DATE DUE

the**facts**

Angina and
Heart Attack

➜ also available in the**facts** series

ADHD, SECOND EDITION
Selikowitz
978-0-19-956503-0 | July 2009

Alzheimer's and other Dementias
Hughes
978-0-19-959655-3 | August 2011

Angina and Heart Attack
Jevon
978-0-19-959928-8 | November 2011

Breast Cancer
Saunders
978-0-19-955869-8 | June 2009

Cosmetic Surgery
Waterhouse
978-0-19-921882-0 | March 2008

Depression, SECOND EDITION
Wasserman
978-0-19-960293-3 | October 2011

Down Syndrome, THIRD EDITION
Selikowitz
978-0-19-923277-2 | May 2008

Epilepsy in Women
Betts
978-0-19-954883-5 | December 2008

Heart Disease
Chenzbraun
978-0-19-958281-5 | August 2010

Infertility
Davies
978-0-19-921769-4 | October 2008

Insomnia and Other Adult Sleep
Problems
Stores
978-0-19-956083-7 | January 2009

Lung Cancer, THIRD EDITION
Falk
978-0-19-956933-5 | October 2009

Obsessive-Compulsive Disorder,
FOURTH EDITION
Rachman
978-0-19-956177-3 | March 2009

Osteoporosis
Black
978-0-19-921589-8 | February 2009

Panic Disorder, THIRD EDITION
Rachman
978-0-19-957469-8 | October 2009

Polycystic Ovary Syndrome
Elsheikh
978-0-19-921368-9 | January 2008

Post-traumatic Stress
Regel
978-0-19-956658-7 | April 2010

Pre-Natal Tests and Ultrasound
Burton
978-0-19-959930-1 | September 2011

Prostate Cancer, SECOND EDITION
Mason
978-0-19-957393-6 | June 2010

Pulmonary Arterial Hypertension
Handler
978-0-19-958292-1 | June 2010

Schizophrenia, THIRD EDITION
Tsuang
978-0-19-960091-5 | August 2011

Sexually Transmitted Infections,
THIRD EDITION
Barlow
978-0-19-959565-5 | March 2011

Sleep Problems in Children and
Adolescents
Stores
978-0-19-929614-9 | November 2008

The Pill and Other Forms of
Hormonal Contraception,
SEVENTH EDITION
Guillebaud
978-0-19-956576-4 | July 2009

the**facts**

Angina and Heart Attack

PHIL JEVON

Resuscitation Officer/Clinical Skills Lead,
Manor Hospital, Walsall, UK

OXFORD
UNIVERSITY PRESS

OXFORD
UNIVERSITY PRESS

Great Clarendon Street, Oxford OX2 6DP

Oxford University Press is a department of the University of Oxford.
It furthers the University's objective of excellence in research, scholarship,
and education by publishing worldwide in

Oxford New York

Auckland Cape Town Dar es Salaam Hong Kong Karachi
Kuala Lumpur Madrid Melbourne Mexico City Nairobi
New Delhi Shanghai Taipei Toronto

With offices in

Argentina Austria Brazil Chile Czech Republic France Greece
Guatemala Hungary Italy Japan Poland Portugal Singapore
South Korea Switzerland Thailand Turkey Ukraine Vietnam

Oxford is a registered trade mark of Oxford University Press
in the UK and in certain other countries

Published in the United States
by Oxford University Press Inc., New York

British Library Cataloguing in Publication Data

Data available

Library of Congress Cataloging in Publication Data

Data available

Typeset in Plantin by Cenveo, Bangalore, India

Printed in Great Britain on acid-free paper by
Clays Ltd, St Ives plc

ISBN 978-0-19-959928-8

10 9 8 7 6 5 4 3 2 1

Whilst every effort has been made to ensure that the contents of this book are as complete, accurate
and up-to-date as possible at the date of writing, Oxford University Press is not able to give any
guarantee or assurance that such is the case. Readers are urged to take appropriately qualified
medical advice in all cases. The information in this book is intended to be useful to the general
reader, but should not be used as a means of self-diagnosis or for the prescription of medication.

Contents

Contributors

Dr Andrew John Hartland, Consultant Chemical Pathologist, Walsall Hospitals NHS Trust, Walsall. UK

Phil Jevon, Resuscitation Officer/Clinical Skills Lead, Manor Hospital, Walsall, UK

Dionne Parsley, Staff Nurse, Cardiology Ward, Walsall Hospitals NHS Trust, Walsall, UK

Emma Simkiss, Senior ECG Technician, Clinical Measurements Department, Walsall Hospitals NHS Trust, Walsall, UK

Dr Fraz Umar MD MRCP, SpR Cardiology Rotation, University Hospital of Coventry and Warwickshire, UK

Simone Waddison, Staff Nurse, Cardiology Ward, Walsall Hospitals NHS Trust, Walsall, UK

Consultant editors

Dr J. Rumi Jaumdally, Consultant Cardiologist, Manor Hospital, Walsall, UK

Dr K. Al-Allaf, Consultant Cardiologist, Manor Hospital, Walsall, UK

1

What is angina and what is a heart attack?

Simone Waddison and Dionne Parsley

> **→ Key points**
>
> - The myocardium (muscle of the heart) needs an adequate blood supply
> - Coronary arteries supply blood to the myocardium
> - Coronary heart disease (CHD) can result in a diminished blood supply to the myocardium
> - Risk factors for CHD include smoking, poor diet and being overweight
> - Angina and a heart attack can result from CHD

Introduction

Coronary heart disease (CHD) is the most common cause of death in both men and women in the UK. There are around 2.6 million people living in the UK with CHD. Each year in the UK, approximately 88,000 deaths are due to CHD. Angina is mainly caused by CHD and 5% of men and 4% of women are living with angina in the UK. If angina is left untreated it can lead to a heart attack or even sudden death. Every six minutes someone in the UK dies from a heart attack.

In this chapter what is angina and what is a heart attack will be discussed. Firstly though, it would be helpful to outline basic anatomy and physiology of the heart and circulation as well as explain what is meant by CHD.

Anatomy and physiology of the heart

Muscular pump

The heart is a muscle that pumps blood around the body. The heart is about the size of the person's fist. It sits in the middle of the chest behind the breast bone (sternum), and is tilted slightly to the left. The heart pumps blood and oxygen to the tissues in the body, and carries away carbon dioxide and other waste products. A system of blood vessels carries blood around the body.

Structure of the heart

The heart is made up of four chambers, two on the left side of the heart and two on the right side of the heart (Fig. 1.1). The two upper chambers are called the atria, and the two lower chambers are called the ventricles. The two sides of the heart are divided by a muscular wall called the septum. The walls of the chambers are made mainly of special heart muscle. The different sections of the heart have to contract in the correct order for the heart to pump blood efficiently with each heartbeat.

A one-way valve system is present in each side of the heart. This means that blood can only travel in one direction through the two chambers on each side of the heart.

Circulation of blood

The right side of the heart receives deoxygenated blood (lacking oxygen) from the body. Deoxygenated blood passes through the right atrium and right ventricle, and is then pumped through the pulmonary artery and to the lungs. Here the blood picks up oxygen, and loses an unwanted gas called carbon dioxide.

Once through the lungs, the blood flows into the left atrium, and then passes into the left ventricle. The heart then contracts and blood is pumped forward into the aorta, which is the main artery supplying the body. Oxygenated blood

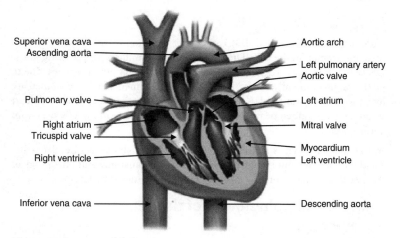

Figure 1.1 Structure of the heart

Reproduced with kind permission of the British Heart Foundation, the copyright owner

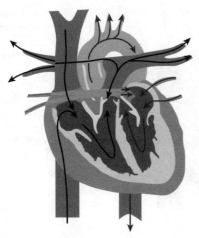

The flow of deoxygenated blood through the right side of the heart is represented by the **dark** line, and the flow of oxygenated blood through the left side of the heart is represented by the **light** line.

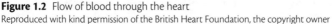

Figure 1.2 Flow of blood through the heart
Reproduced with kind permission of the British Heart Foundation, the copyright owner

is then carried through the arteries to all of the body's tissues. Oxygen and other nutrients then pass into the body's cells where they are used to carry out the body's essential functions.

The blood then travels back to the heart. The blood goes from the very small blood vessels (capillaries) into the veins, which then join to form larger veins. The larger veins then deliver blood back to the right side of the heart.

When the heart relaxes in between each heartbeat, blood from the veins refills the right side of the heart, and blood from the lungs refills the left side of the heart.

The coronary circulation

Like any other muscle in the body, the heart muscle (myocardium) needs a good blood supply. This supply of blood comes from the coronary arteries which start from the beginning of the aorta. The coronary arteries spread across the outer of the myocardium, giving a continuous supply of fresh blood to the heart muscle.

The right coronary artery mainly supplies the muscle of the right ventricle. The left coronary artery splits into two and supplies the rest of the heart muscle. The main coronary arteries divide into many smaller branches to supply all the heart muscle. After supplying the myocardium the blood flows back into the coronary veins.

The coronary arteries receive about 5% of the blood pumped by the heart, despite the heart representing a small amount of total body weight. This large blood supply shows the importance of the heart to body function.

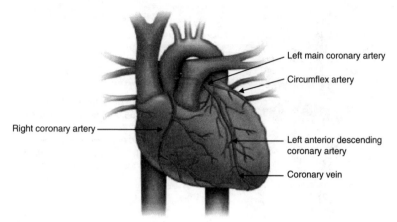

Left main coronary artery

Circumflex artery

Right coronary artery

Left anterior descending coronary artery

Coronary vein

Figure 1.3 Coronary circulation
Reproduced with kind permission of the British Heart Foundation, the copyright owner

Conduction system in the heart

The heart beats by following a series of electrical signals that makes the muscles in each chamber of the heart contract (pump) in a certain order. The sequence of these signals is as follows (also see diagram below):

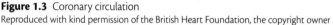

- The heart's own built in pacemaker controls the heart rate. This is located in the right atrium, and is called the sinoatrial node (SA node). The SA node discharges an electrical impulse at regular intervals, usually about 60–80 a minute at rest, and faster during exercise. Every impulse spreads across the right and left atria, which makes them contract. When this happens, blood is pumped through the one-way valves into the ventricles.

- The impulse then reaches a 'junction box' located in the lower right atrium. This is called the atrioventricular node (AV node). The impulse is delayed slightly here. The tissue between the atria and ventricles does not conduct the impulse. However, a thin band of conducting tissue called the 'Bundle of His' operates like wires and passes the impulse from the AV node to the ventricles.

- The Bundle of His then splits in two, forming the left bundle branch and the right bundle branch. These carry the electrical impulse through the ventricles. This then makes the ventricles contract which pumps blood through the one-way valves into the pulmonary artery and the aorta.

- The sequence will then start again for the next heartbeat.

Coronary heart disease (CHD)

CHD is caused by a gradual accumulation of fatty deposits in the linings of the walls of the arteries and blood vessels (Fig. 1.5a) that deliver blood to the heart muscle. This condition is known as atherosclerosis and the fatty deposits are

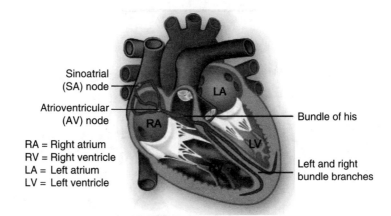

Figure 1.4 Conduction system in the heart
Reproduced with permission from the Texas Heart Institute http://www.texasheartinstitute.org/HIC/anatomy/conduct.cfm

called atheroma or plaque. Atherosclerosis can result in a reduced blood flow to the heart muscle. Progressively the arteries can become very narrow and hard therefore reducing the amount of blood and oxygen delivered to the heart muscle (Fig.1.5b). This can cause chest pain or discomfort and is known as angina. A plaque can also rupture from the side of the artery wall causing clots to form which can partially or totally occlude the artery (Fig. 1.5c). When this occurs blood cannot deliver oxygen to the heart muscle and the heart is unable to function properly. This is called a heart attack and emergency medical assistance is required.

Incidence of CHD

The incidence of heart attacks in the UK has decreased over the last three decades, which is mainly put down to changes in lifestyle and behaviours. In Scotland, the incidence of heart attacks has decreased by 25% between 2000–2009 in both men and women.

The prevalence of heart attacks increases greatly with age, with incidence also being higher in men than in women. However, the difference between the sexes decreases with age. It is estimated that there are around 62,000 heart attacks in English men and 39,000 in English women every year, and 8,000 heart attacks in Scottish men and 5,000 in Scottish women every year.

It is estimated that in 2009 the incidence of angina was the highest in Scotland and the lowest in England for both men and women. Overall in the UK, incidence rate were 75% higher in men compared to women. The incidence rate generally increases with age, and the highest rate is between the ages of 65–74 years for both men and women. Using these rates, it can be estimated that there are nearly 28,000 new cases of angina every year in the UK.

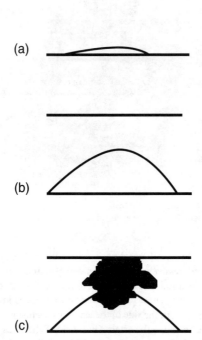

(a)

(b)

(c)

Figure 1.5 Coronary heart disease; a. The early formation of atherosclerosis plaque; b. A mature plaque; c. A ruptured plaque with the formation of a blood clot

From age and sex specific incidence estimates, it can be said that there are around 1 million men and around 500,000 women living in the UK who have suffered a heart attack. A large number of these people, around 900,000 are aged less than 75 years. However, the incidence of angina is higher than the incidence of people who have suffered a heart attack. There are around 1.2 million men and around 900,000 women living in the UK with angina, with over 1.2 million of these people being aged less than 75 years.

The incidence of CHD in the UK increases with age and is higher in men than in women. In the UK there are around 1.6 million men and around 1 million women living with CHD, with 1.6 million of these people being aged less than 75 years.

Evidence has shown that certain minority ethnic groups have a higher incidence of CHD than other groups. It has been found that in general, all South Asian groups have higher rates or conditions including angina and heart attacks, compared to the general population. However, Chinese men and women have shown to have lower rates of these conditions than the general population.

Black Caribbean men (but not women) have a significantly lower incidence of angina and heart attacks than the general population.

Death rates from CHD

Cardiovascular disease (CVD) is the main cause of death in the UK and accounts for almost 191,000 deaths each year, which is one in three of all deaths. Nearly half (46%) of deaths from CVD are from CHD. In 2008 about one in five men and about one in eight women died from CHD.

CHD is the most common cause of premature death in the UK. Premature death is defined as death before the age of 75. About one fifth (18%) of premature deaths in men and one in ten (9%) of premature deaths in women were from CHD in 2008, causing about 28,000 premature deaths in the UK in this year.

Since the early 1970s, death rates from CVD in the UK have been falling. In recent years, death rates from CHD have been falling more slowly in younger age groups and fastest in those aged over 55. Between 1998 and 2008 CHD death rates for men aged 55–64 years in the UK fell by 49%, compared to 26% for men aged 35–44 years. In women, there was a fall in death rates of 55% in those aged 55–64 years, and the death rates in those aged 35–44 years barely changed.

It can be said that more than half (58%) of the decline in death rates from CHD during the 1980s and 1990s can be put down to people adopting a healthier life-style, largely from people quitting or not smoking at all. The rest of the decline (42%) can be put down to improvements in the care of people with CHD.

There are differences in the number of death rates depending on where in the UK you live. Death rates from CHD are the highest in Scotland and North of England, lowest in the South of England, and midway in Wales and Northern Ireland. The rate of premature deaths for men living in Scotland is 63% higher than in the South West of England and 100% higher for women.

There are also differences in death rates from CHD depending upon social class. Death rates in 2001–2003 were highest in the lowest social groups, and lowest in the highest social groups. This variation was more remarkable in women than in men, with the death rate in women with routine jobs five times higher than those with managerial or professional jobs.

Risk factors for CHD

The risk factors for CHD are discussed in detail in the next chapter. Some of the main risk factors will be briefly mentioned here:

Smoking: smoking considerably increases the risk of CHD. It has been found that death rates from CHD are around 60% higher in smokers, and around

80% higher in heavy smokers, compared to non-smokers. A study found that around half of all regular smokers will eventually be killed through this habit.

In Great Britain, about 21% of adults smoke cigarettes. Younger age groups tend to smoke the most, and those aged over 60 years tend to smoke the least. Smoking has been declining since the 1970s and 1980s in the UK, and it is hoped that the ban on smoking in public places will reduce the rates of young people who smoke.

Poor diet: a poor diet can increase the risk of developing a chronic condition, including CHD. When people consume a poor diet and take on more energy than is used, the results can be weight gain and obesity. Eating foods that are high in saturated fats can raise cholesterol levels, food high in salt can increase blood pressure, and low intakes of fibre, fruit and vegetables can lead to a greater risk of developing CHD.

In the UK, it has been found that average salt intake is above the recommended amount of 6g per day, with the average consumption being 9–10g per day for men, and 7g per day for women. Average consumption of fibre is also lower than the recommended amount, at 14g per day compared to the recommendation of 18g per day. Also, only around one third of men and women consume the recommended five portions of fruit and vegetables per day.

Physical inactivity: people who are physically active are at a lower risk of developing CHD. To achieve the maximum benefit, exercise should be regular and aerobic. Exercise should involve the use of the larger muscle groups steadily and rhythmically to increase the heart rate and breathing significantly. The recommended amount of exercise for adults is 30 minutes of physical activity at least 5 days a week.

Alcohol consumption: moderate alcohol consumption (one or two drinks a day) does not increase the risk of CHD. However, it is estimated that 2% of CHD in men in developed countries is due to alcohol. Despite this, the effect of alcohol consumption in women in developed countries is said to be positive, as when no alcohol is consumed there is a 3% increase in CHD. It is advised by the Government that regular consumption of three to four units a day for men, and two to three units a day for women will not lead to significant health risk. However, consuming over these levels is not advised.

Reducing the risk

The incidence of CHD can be reduced when people make small changes to their lifestyle. For people who already have the condition, making the changes can help to keep their heart healthy and reduce the risk of future problems. These changes include:

◆ Stopping smoking
◆ Controlling high blood pressure

◆ Reducing your cholesterol level

◆ Being physically active

◆ Achieving and maintaining a healthy weight

◆ Controlling your blood glucose if you have diabetes

◆ Eating a healthy balanced diet, and only drinking moderate amounts of alcohol.

What is angina?

The term angina is pain or tightness in the chest (from the Greek word *agkhone*—strangling). Angina is the most common symptom of CHD and it can be divided into two main types: stable or unstable angina.

Stable angina

Stable angina usually occurs on exertion and is where the myocardial (heart muscle) demand for blood (and oxygen) exceeds the supply. The heart muscle receives its blood supply from two large blood vessels known as the left and right coronary arteries (see above). At rest the heart muscles can cope with the supply of blood that is being delivered through the coronary arteries. When exercising, however, such as climbing the stairs, the heart muscle is working harder resulting in an increased demand for blood (and oxygen). But due to the narrow and hard coronary arteries there is insufficient supply of blood to the heart muscle (Fig. 1.5b) and the heart is unable to work efficiently. This can lead to the symptoms of stable angina which can vary from one individual to another. Some people may describe having central chest pain that is heavy, crushing or tight in nature whilst others may experience a dull ache. The pain may or may not radiate to other areas of the body such as the neck, jaw, shoulders, back, stomach or the arm, usually the left one. Angina pain can also be known to be associated with shortness of breath and sweating. Other symptoms may include dizziness, belching, nausea, tired, and restlessness. Angina can also be brought on by strong emotions, cold weather or after eating a heavy meal; these are known as triggers. Angina is usually relieved at rest or generally responds to medication so is usually short-lived, lasting five minutes or less.

Incidence of angina

	Black Caribbean	Indian	Pakistani	Bangladeshi	Chinese	Irish	General Population
Men (%)	1.9	5.4	2.9	3.9	1.8	4.8	5.3
Women (%)	2.2	1.7	1.5	1.3	0.4	2.9	3.9

It can be seen from the above table that the highest incidence rate of angina is amongst Indian men, which is nearly as high as the rate for the whole of the general population. It can also be seen that in all ethnic groups, except for Black Caribbean, incidence rates are lower for women compared to men.

Unstable angina

Unstable angina usually occurs at rest and can wake you from sleep. It gradually gets worse over time. It is caused when atherosclerosis plaque ruptures. Red blood cells responsible for clotting then collect on the surface of the plaque causing a large blood clot to form (Fig. 1.5c). This can then block off the coronary artery and trigger the symptoms of unstable angina. The symptoms may not respond to treatment and this is a medical emergency because it can progress to a heart attack if left untreated. The symptoms of unstable angina are similar to those of stable angina but they can last for twenty to thirty minutes or even longer. It may not respond to treatment and can occur without any triggers. If you feel that you or somebody else is having an unstable angina attack then dial 999 and ask for an ambulance. It is important to be admitted to hospital for further tests and treatment.

Diagnosis

The doctor may be able to diagnose angina from the symptoms that you describe. So it is important to answer questions as accurately as possible. Your family and lifestyle history can identify if you are at an increased risk of developing angina. Blood tests can identify if there is too much cholesterol in your blood which can form plaque, or if you are diabetic because excess sugar in the blood can damage the blood vessels. An electrocardiogram (ECG) is a test that looks at the heart rhythm and can identify if the heart is not getting enough blood. This is a simple test to perform and involves placing some sticky electrode dots on the chest, arms and legs and connecting the ECG machine to them to monitor the heartbeat. Another possible test used to diagnose angina is an exercise tolerance test (ETT) where you are attached to an ECG machine and you will need to exercise either on a stationary bike or a treadmill. The test identifies how much exercise the heart can deal with before the symptoms of angina are triggered. These are just some of the investigations used to diagnose angina. A more detailed review is provided in Chapter 4.

Treatment for angina

There are different treatment options for stable and unstable angina, but people that are diagnosed with either condition usually receive medication for it. The doctor involved with your care will prescribe the most suitable drugs for you as not all drugs are suitable for all due to side effects, allergy, current medication and past medical history. Some of the more widely used drugs may include nitrates, anti-platelets e.g. aspirin, beta-blockers, calcium channel blockers, angiotensin-converting enzyme (ACE) inhibitors and statins.

What is a heart attack

In the UK there is a high number of deaths that result from heart disease and most of these are caused by a heart attack. One in five men and one in seven women die from heart disease. A heart attack is a serious medical emergency and one in three people die before reaching hospital.

The medical term for a heart attack is a myocardial infarction (MI) or acute coronary syndrome (ACS). A heart attack can occur in people with CHD. This is where the coronary arteries that deliver blood to the heart muscle become narrow and hard due to atherosclerosis plaque. A heart attack occurs when the plaque becomes unstable or ulcerates and ruptures causing a blood clot to form. This will then totally or partially suddenly block off the blood supply to the heart starving it of oxygen. This can cause irreversible damage to the heart muscle if left untreated.

Types of heart attack

There are two main types of heart attack where damage to the heart muscle occurs. These are known as ST segment elevation myocardial infarction (STEMI) and non-ST segment elevation myocardial infarction (NSTEMI). They are classified this way by measurement of the electrical heart rhythm that is recorded on an ECG. The ST segment identifies the level of damage that has occurred during the heart attack. Usually the higher the ST segment, the greater amount of damage has occurred to the heart muscle.

- *STEMI*: this occurs when the ruptured atheroma plaque and blood clot completely blocks the coronary artery interrupting the blood supply to the heart muscle for a prolonged period (Fig. 1.5c). This can cause a large amount of damage to the heart muscle and is the most serious type of heart attack. It can lead to sudden death and urgent medical assistance is required. There is a significant ST change on the ECG.

- *NSTEMI*: this is caused by a partial or temporary blockage of the coronary artery by the plaque and blood clot so interrupting the blood supply for a limited period of time. Damage to the heart muscle still occurs, but much smaller by comparison to that of a STEMI. There is no ST change on the ECG, but this is still an emergency and medical assistance is required.

Symptoms

The symptoms of a heart attack can vary from one individual to another. The most common symptom is central chest pain. It can feel like heavy crushing pressure, tightness or squeezing on the chest, or even a dull ache or discomfort. It can last for at least twenty minutes and continue for several hours. The pain is not relieved at rest and may move to other parts of the body such as:

- The neck
- The jaw

- The shoulders
- The stomach
- The back
- The arms (usually the left one)

The following symptoms may also be associated:

- Feeling sick or vomiting
- Shortness of breath
- Sweating
- Fear and anxiety
- Light headedness
- Feeling generally unwell

There are reported cases in which people have not experienced chest pain at all, for example some women, some of the elderly and some people that are known to have diabetes. Therefore you should not rely purely on experiencing chest pain to determine whether or not you have had a heart attack, but instead to look at the overall pattern of symptoms that you have and seek emergency help by calling 999 for an ambulance.

Diagnosis

If it is suspected that you are having a heart attack you will need to be admitted into hospital, usually into a specialist coronary care unit. Diagnosis of a heart attack usually involves taking a medical history, a physical examination and performing some diagnostic tests. The 12 lead ECG is one of the first tests that you will have and it measures the electrical activity of the heart. It can identify if a heart attack is in progress or has already occurred and also the type of heart attack that you have had. Another test that helps to diagnose a heart attack is a troponin blood test. This is usually taken around twelve hours after your symptoms started. Healthy heart cells contain enzymes which are proteins that regulate the rate of chemical reaction in the body. If there is damage to the heart the cells will die and enzymes will slowly leak into your blood. The blood test therefore detects raised enzyme levels due to the death of specialist heart cells. The level of these enzymes can also determine the size of the heart attack. A heart attack can be confirmed by these tests alone—your symptoms, ECG result and troponin blood result. Whilst you are in hospital your consultant will advise you to have further tests to fully assess the condition of your heart and to help determine further treatment. These will be discussed further in Chapter 7.

Treatment after a heart attack

Once the diagnosis of a heart attack has been made treatment starts straight away. The primary goal is to restore normal blood flow to the damaged area of the heart as soon as possible and to preserve the function of the rest of the heart. The main treatment options are usually medication or surgical intervention:

◆ *Medication*: this is by drugs known as thrombolytics or 'clot busting' drugs. It is injected into you and given in a one off dose ideally within the first few hours following a heart attack. Thrombolytics drugs destroy a substance called fibrin which is a toughened fibre around a blood clot holding it together. This then enables the clot to be dissolved. You may also be given additional blood thinning medication to minimise the risk of further clots developing.

◆ *Coronary angioplasty*: an intervention that is also used for unstable angina and involves passing a wire into the blood vessels to the coronary arteries under guided X-ray and widening the artery to improve blood flow to the heart. A wire mesh may also be inserted into the artery to keep it open.

Your doctor will also prescribe you a combination of medication to enable your heart to work efficiently, to reduce further complications and to control your symptoms.

Complications of a heart attack

The location of the heart attack determines how the heart muscle functions afterwards. If blockage occurs to the artery supplying blood to the front part of the heart it affects the left side of the heart which is responsible for pumping blood all around the body. This is most dangerous type of heart attack and sudden death can occur. Heart failure can also occur as a result because the muscle is badly damaged and is unable to pump blood around the body. If blockage occurs to the artery supplying blood to the right side of the heart it affects the part of the heart that is responsible for the electrical activity that keeps the heart beating. As a result of this abnormal heart rhythms can occur where the heart can beat too quickly, too slow or irregularly.

Further reading

British Heart Foundation (2010a) *Living with a heart condition.* [online]. London: BHF. www.bhf.org.uk.

British Heart Foundation (2010b) *Coronary heart disease statistics 2010: Chapter 1–2.* [online]. London: BHF. www.bhf.org.uk.

British Heart Foundation (2010c) *Cardiovascular (heart and circulatory disease).* [online]. London: BHF. www.bhf.org.uk.

2

What are the causes of ischaemic heart disease?

Andrew Hartland

 Key points

- There is usually not just one cause for a person's heart disease, but the culmination of a number of risk factors
- The commonest risk factors are: smoking, high cholesterol, diabetes, high blood pressure, being overweight, stress and heredity (similar problems running in the family)
- Smoking and having a high cholesterol makes up more than two-thirds of the risk of developing heart disease
- Having diabetes increases the dangerousness of the other risk factors, so diabetics usually need medication to lower their blood pressure and cholesterol

Smoking

Smoking causes around 25,000 deaths from heart and circulatory disease each year. Around one in five premature deaths from heart and circulatory disease are linked to smoking.

All the ways by which smoking causes heart disease are not known. However, smoking is known to make blood more likely to clot, and a blood clot is the usual cause of a heart attack. It also increases blood pressure. Smoking lowers the amount of HDL (good cholesterol) making atherosclerosis (the build up of fatty substances on the lining of arteries) more likely. It damages the lining of blood vessels and heart attacks are more likely if the lining to the arteries of the heart are damaged. By all these ways, smoking increases the risk of heart disease.

The risk of smoking depends on how much a person smokes (how many cigarettes a day) and for how long they have been a smoker.

No form of tobacco smoking is safe. Smoking a pipe or cigars can be as dangerous as smoking cigarettes.

Most of the risk of a heart attack due to smoking can be removed if the person stops smoking. The risk reduces much quicker than most people think. The risk of a heart attack can be reduced within a few months of stopping smoking, even in someone who has been a heavy smoker for many years.

Women who smoke and use oral contraceptives greatly increase their risk of coronary heart disease and stroke compared with non-smoking women who use oral contraceptives.

Techniques to stop smoking do work. More people are successful at stopping smoking if helped by a smoking cessation programme or by using nicotine patches. However, all ways of stopping smoking need will-power.

Frequently Asked Questions

Q: I am a smoker. I have heard that if I switch to low-tar cigarettes, this will be sufficient?

A: No, it is preferable to give up smoking completely. It has also been shown that smokers of low tar cigarettes actually inhale just as much tar and nicotine as smokers of standard cigarettes. If you switch to low tar cigarettes, you are likely to breathe in more heavily and also to take extra puffs on the cigarette.

Q: I have already had a heart attack so is it really worth giving up smoking? Isn't the damage already done?

A: Yes, giving up smoking will reduce the risk of having another heart attack. In fact, smokers who manage to give up smoking for 15 years have a similar risk of a heart attack to someone who has never smoked.

Poor diet

Eating a lot of high-fat, sugary or salty foods increases the risk of heart disease. It raises blood pressure, increases cholesterol and causes weight gain.

Eating five portions of fruit and veg a day reduces the risk of heart disease. The exact reasons are not fully known, but an important factor is probable that fruit and vegetables contain a lot of nutrients called 'anti-oxidants'. These seem to lower the amount of chemicals called 'free radicals' in the blood, leading to less fatty build up inside arteries (atherosclerosis). They also seem to protect the lining of blood vessels from damage, which may lower blood pressure.

A healthy way of eating is for your usual diet to be a balance of protein (lean meat, fish, dairy products or vegetarian alternatives if vegetarian), unsaturated fats, carbohydrates (starchy foods like bread and pasta), fruit and vegetables. It should be low in saturated fat, salt and sugar.

The principles of healthy eating for the heart are:

1) Eat regular meals (and no snacking)

2) Cut down on sugary food and drinks

3) Reduce the amount of saturated fat

4) Eat at least five portions of fruit and veg a day

5) Cut down on salt. Don't add salt to your food

6) Reduce your alcohol

Eating regular meals

Starchy foods (such as potatoes, bread, cereals, pasta) release their energy slowly, as they need to be digested first. This helps you feel satisfied for longer. It also helps keep blood sugar levels constant. This prevents the sugar dips which can cause hunger pangs.

Cut down on high-sugar food and drinks

Sugary food and drinks are high in calories. The body turns the sugar calories that are not used into fat, causing weight gain.

Sugar is absorbed quickly from the gut into the blood. This causes blood glucose levels to rise quickly after a meal and then drop again. This rapid drop can make a person feel hungry again.

Sugary drinks (fizzy drinks, cordials) are high in calories but low in nutrients. They add to your calorie count without making you feel full.

Reduce the amount of fat in your diet

We all eat much more fat than we need.

Reducing saturated fat (fatty meats, biscuits, pastry, full-fat dairy products) lowers cholesterol.

Eat five portions of fruit and vegetables every day

This has been proven to reduce blood pressure and prevent heart disease.

Cut down on salt

The more salt you eat, the higher your blood pressure is likely to be.

So, don't add salt to meals or when cooking and choose low-salt food options when available.

Reduce your alcohol

Although there is some evidence that very moderate alcohol consumption (2 units a day) may have a protective effect, reducing the risk of heart disease in men over 40 years of age and women who have gone through the menopause, this information must be taken with caution. Any benefits from alcohol soon turn into negatives when higher levels of alcohol are consumed. Also, the benefits of alcohol only seem to work if the alcohol is consumed during a meal.

Remember, alcohol is very high in calories, and weight gain increases the risk of heart disease. Therefore, drink alcohol in moderation, no more than 2 units a day, as part of a meal.

Oily fish

Some studies have shown that eating oily fish regularly can help reduce the risk of heart disease, but this has not been shown by all studies looking at this. It is thought that omega-3 fatty acids, which are found in large amounts in oily fish, help keep the heartbeat regular, reduce the levels of triglycerides (fats found in the blood) reducing the likelihood of fatty build up inside arteries (atherosclerosis) and helping prevent blood clots.

The British Heart Foundation recommends eating oily fish (two portions a week).

Oily fish include fresh tuna, salmon, trout, mackerel and herring. Try to avoid smoked fish, which is usually high in salt.

High cholesterol

Having high cholesterol is a major risk factor for developing heart disease.

Cholesterol is a fatty substance found in the blood. Most of the cholesterol in the blood does not come directly from what we have eaten, but has been made by the body itself, in the liver. Nevertheless, what we eat can affect how much cholesterol is in our blood. Eating foods high in saturated fat can lead to having too much blood cholesterol.

Although some foods contain cholesterol (such as eggs, liver, kidney and some seafood), eating these foods does not usually cause high blood cholesterol. It is more important to reduce the amount of saturated fat eaten and replace with poly or monounsaturated fat.

Cholesterol is carried in the blood by proteins in particles called lipoproteins. There are two types of lipoproteins:

Low Density Lipoproteins (LDL): These can be harmful, because they can be taken up by the lining of blood vessels, causing a fatty build up on the inside of arteries (a process called atherosclerosis). These build ups (or plaques) can narrow the blood vessels, reducing the amount of blood that can get through. If this happens in the blood vessels supplying the heart muscle, this causes a cramp-like sensation called angina. If the plaque becomes damaged, a blood clot can form across the damaged plaque blocking the blood vessel completely. If this happens in one of the arteries supplying the heart muscle, this is called a heart attack (or myocardial infarction, often shortened to MI). Too much LDL is harmful and sometimes this type of cholesterol is called 'bad cholesterol'.

High Density Lipoproteins (HDL): This can be protective (and is often called 'good cholesterol'). It is protective because, if a HDL particle travelling in the blood collides with a plaque, it takes away some of the cholesterol from the plaque, making it smaller.

Most people have too much LDL ('bad cholesterol') and not enough HDL ('good cholesterol').

LDL can be reduced by cutting down on saturated fat and replacing in the diet with mono or polyunsaturated fat. There is also some evidence that eating substances called 'plant sterols' and 'stanols' can reduce LDL. These plant sterols/stanols are found in certain margarines, spreads and yoghurts.

HDL cholesterol can be increased by regular physical activity (exercise). It can also be raised by moderate alcohol intakes—but not more than 2 units of alcohol per day is advised!

LDL cholesterol can also be reduced (and HDL raised) by medication. The most effective type of medications for lowering LDL cholesterol are called statins. There are a number of different statins that can be prescribed (for example, simvastatin, atorvastatin, pravastatin, resouvastatin). Statins have been scientifically proven to reduce heart disease and the risk of heart attack. They are advised for all patients at high risk of a heart attack, and should be taken life long by patients who have heart disease to help stop the heart disease getting worse. Statins are amongst the most commonly prescribed medication in the world and have been widely prescribed for many years. Side effects from statins are so few that simvastatin can be bought over-the-counter at chemist shops without prescription. Some people do get side effects, the commonest being a muscle ache, but most people take statins without any problems at all.

Fibrates are another type of medication given to lower blood cholesterol. They do lower LDL cholesterol but not as effectively as statins. Fibrates are very effective at lowering a type of blood fat called triglyceride. In most people triglycerides are not a major cause of atherosclerosis, but it is known that having high triglycerides is a risk factor for developing heart disease. Fibrates are sometimes used if a person has side effects with statins.

Eating omega-3 fatty acids (in oily fish) also helps lower triglycerides.

Some people still have too much blood cholesterol despite a good diet.

Some people have very high blood cholesterol due to a genetic condition. There are a number of these conditions. They are all rare, but the commonest is called Familial Hypercholesterolaemia (FH). Common to all of these is that heart problems usually run in the family, and usually occur at a relatively young age. Blood tests can be done to investigate whether a person has one of these conditions. Treatment is usually with tablets.

We still do not know how low we need to get someone's blood cholesterol in order to reduce the risk of heart disease as much as possible. Currently, the agreed target for someone treated with medication is to reduce cholesterol to less that 4.0 mmol/L and the amount of LDL cholesterol to less than 2.0 mmol/L.

If someone is having their first ever blood test for cholesterol it is often useful if the patient has a fasted sample taken (this means that he/she has nothing to eat for the 8 hours before the blood test. This usually means having the blood test taken in the morning, with the patients having missed breakfast, including having no milk or sugar in tea or coffee). This is because a fasting sample is need to accurately assess triglycerides. After this, most blood tests for blood cholesterol do not require the patient to have fasted (fasting makes hardly any difference to the cholesterol levels).

Overweight

Being overweight increases the risk of heart disease in a number of ways. It increases blood pressure and cholesterol levels. It also greatly increases the chances of becoming diabetic.

> Having a body mass index (BMI) greater that 30 kg/m^2 reduces life expectancy by 2–4 years.
>
> Having a BMI greater than 40 kg/m^2 reduces life expectancy by more than 8 years, which is comparable to the risk due to smoking. Heart problems are the major cause of these early deaths.

Having too much visceral fat is believed to be the main reason why being overweight causes health problems such as type 2 diabetes, high blood pressure and heart disease. Visceral fat is the fat which lines the outside of organs such as the heart, the liver and the kidneys. Visceral fat sends out chemical signals which can affect blood vessels and the body's metabolism, leading to a high blood pressure and a raised cholesterol. Usually, the more overweight someone is, the more visceral fat they have.

Waist circumference is a good indicator of visceral fat and so is also a marker of heart risk. If you are a man and your waist circumference is greater than

40 inches, or you are a woman with a waist circumference of more than 35 inches you are at increased risk of heart disease and would benefit from losing weight. Waist circumference should be measured (not taken from clothes size!) by placing a tape measure around you waist, just above the hip bones, while standing. Measure your waist just after you breathe out.

Eating a healthy diet, reducing weight (if overweight) and exercising regularly have been shown to reduce heart disease.

Stress

Although stress is not thought to be a direct risk factor for heart disease, the ways people cope with stress can contribute to the development of heart problems. Many people cope with stress by smoking, drinking alcohol or over-eating. All of these are risk factors for developing heart disease.

Some studies have shown that being depressed increases the risk of heart disease.

If a person has heart disease and feels very anxious or under a lot of stress, the resulting increase in heart rate can bring on symptoms like angina.

How we cope with stress is important in preventing heart disease. Eating a balanced diet and exercising regularly have been shown to help manage stress and increase positive mood and wellbeing. Yoga and other relaxation techniques have also been shown to be useful at managing anxiety.

It is important to identify situations which cause anxiety and avoid them, if possible.

Hereditary

A tendency towards heart disease seems to be hereditary. This means that children whose parents have heart problems may be more likely to develop them.

A family history of diabetes, high blood pressure or high cholesterol may increase the risk of heart disease.

A number of genes have been associated with high blood pressure, heart disease and stroke in large population-based studies. However, the influence of individual genes on individual people is not well understood. At present, these is no specific genetic test for predicting future heart disease.

There are some genetic causes for having a high cholesterol. These can be tested for by genetic blood tests. The commonest is a condition called Familial Hypercholesterolaemia (FH). Blood cholesterol levels found in people with FH are much higher than are found in the general population. Tablets called statins are very effective at lowering blood cholesterol, even if the cause is genetic.

Although we cannot change our genes, we can reduce the risk of heart disease by eating healthily, exercising regularly and avoiding tobacco.

Hypertension

Blood pressure is the pressure of blood in your arteries, the blood vessels which carry blood from the heart to the rest of the body.

When the blood is forced into the arteries as the heart beats, the blood pressure is highest. When the heart is filling (or resting) between heartbeats the blood pressure is lowest.

When a person has their blood pressure measured two readings are taken. The first is the highest blood pressure (as the heart is beating). This is called the systolic pressure (systole being a name for a heartbeat). The second is the lowest blood pressure (between beats). This is called the diastolic pressure. These blood pressure measurements are measured in units called millimetres of mercury (mmHg).

A typical systolic blood pressure may be 130 mmHg. A typical diastolic blood pressure may be 80 mmHg. This would be written as 130/80, and described as '130 over 80'.

Having high blood pressure, or hypertension, means having a blood pressure which is consistently above a level which is considered healthy. Having a high blood pressure is a risk factor for heart disease and heart failure. There remains some uncertainty about what levels constitute a high blood pressure, but most experts agree that if a person has coronary heart disease, angina or has had a heart attack or a stroke, their blood pressure should be less than 130/80 mmHg. Sometimes a lower blood pressure target is set, depending on a person's medical problems.

Hypertension does not usually have an identifiable cause. Known risk factors for developing hypertension include: being overweight, not enough physical exercise, drinking too much alcohol and too much salt in the diet.

Anxiety can raise blood pressure. Some people become anxious when they are about to have their blood pressure measured, which can result in misleadingly high readings. This is often called the 'White coat' syndrome (as the person's blood pressure rises as soon as they see the white coat of a doctor). There are ways around this to enable a more representative blood pressure reading to be obtained. Taking a series of readings over the space of a few weeks can often help. Alternatively, there are simple devices which can be supplied from hospitals which will monitor blood pressure over a 24 hour period.

Diabetes

Diabetes is a condition where the amount of sugar (glucose) in the blood is higher than it should be.

Blood glucose comes from the food we digest. We also store glucose as a substance called carbohydrate. This is usually stored in the liver, but other organs can also store carbohydrate. The liver releases its stored sugar when blood sugar levels are low.

After a meal, the blood glucose rises as the food is digested and absorbed into the body. The body produces a hormone called insulin. Insulin allows cells to take up glucose from the blood. Once taken up, cells use the glucose to produce energy. Therefore, insulin helps keep our blood glucose levels fairly constant.

Diabetes occurs when a person either cannot make enough insulin, or alternatively, the insulin does not work as well as it should.

There are two types of diabetes:

Type 1 diabetes: This occurs when a person cannot make insulin. It usually comes on in childhood or as a young adult. The only treatment is to give insulin (to replace the insulin which is not being made).

Type 2 diabetes: This usually begins by the person's insulin not working as well as it should. This type of diabetes is the commonest seen in the UK. Eight out of ten people in the UK who have diabetes have type 2 diabetes. Why the insulin works less well is not fully known but being overweight and not having enough physical exercise are strong risk factors. In many cases, this type of diabetes does not cause any symptoms (it usually does not cause thirst or excessive urine production) but it can be dangerous if the blood glucoses are not controlled. This type of diabetes usually develops over many years and usually begins after the age of 40, although younger people are beginning to develop type 2 diabetes, especially if they are overweight.

Diabetes increases the risk of developing heart disease. High blood glucose levels affect artery walls, encouraging fatty deposits to build up. Having diabetes can also increase blood pressure and cholesterol levels. It also increases the effect of some other risk factors such as smoking and being overweight.

The chances of developing diabetes can be reduced by keeping to a healthy diet, avoiding becoming overweight and exercising regularly.

For those with diabetes, it is very important to control blood sugar levels, blood pressure and cholesterol levels. This reduces the risk of heart disease.

Most diabetics will need to take a tablet called a statin to lower their cholesterol and reduce their risk of heart disease.

Role of gender, age and ethnicity
Gender

Life expectancy is lower for men than women, and the increased risk of heart disease in men is an important factor.

Men are statistically more likely to smoke and drink too much alcohol, both risk factors for heart disease. Also the female hormone oestrogen has a protective effect on the heart, partly by reducing cholesterol level. This means that heart problems usually occur at a younger age in men (as much as 10 years earlier on average) than in women.

However, it is not all good news for women. Certain risk factors can be more dangerous in women than in men. Diabetes increases the risk of heart disease in women more than in men. It also removes some of the heart disease protection given by oestrogen (for example, although heart disease usually occurs at a younger age in men than in women, having diabetes removes this advantage in women). Also, women who smoke are twice as likely to have a heart attack as men who smoke. In addition, the menstrual cycle affects tobacco withdrawal symptoms, sometimes making nicotine replacement less effective.

> Although the most common symptom of a heart attack is dull central chest pain or chest tightness, women are more likely than men to instead experience more unusual symptoms such as excessive tiredness, disturbed sleep or breathlessness. This can hinder diagnosis.

Age

The risk of heart disease, as with many illnesses, becomes greater the older we get. Most risk factors such as smoking, having diabetes, high blood pressure or high cholesterol contribute slowly to the development of heart disease over many years. Heart disease in someone under 40 years old remains unusual in the UK.

Ethnicity

No ethnic group is immune to heart disease, which remains a major cause of illness and death in almost all races. However, as the causes of heart disease are a combination of genes and environment, it is not surprising that genetic differences across ethnic groups are seen. For example, people of South Asian origin appear to be at particularly high risk of heart disease, both because they seem to be more likely to have risk factors such as diabetes and high blood pressure and also these risk factors seem to be more dangerous in this group. However, preventative measures can be effective in any racial group.

Risk

There has been a lot of discussion about 'risk factors' and 'risk'. Many of us will know of someone who has smoked 20 cigarettes a day for over 50 years and is alive and well, while someone else who lives a healthy lifestyle has heart problems at a young age. However, in general, people who smoke are more likely to get heart problems, and at a younger age, than people who don't. This is what is meant when we say that something is a risk factor—it makes heart disease more likely.

It is useful to have an idea how much more likely (or how great a risk factor) something is. Buying 50 lottery tickets instead of one increases the chances (or risk) of winning the lottery, but only very slightly, whereas buying 50 raffle tickets for a raffle where only 100 tickets are sold greatly increases the chances of winning (but doesn't guarantee it).

In terms of heart disease, there are a number of different methods for calculating a person's risk based on their age, and risk factors such as smoking, blood pressure and diabetes. A person is considered to be at high risk if their 10 year risk of developing a heart problem is 20% or more, which means that they have a 2 in 10 chance or more of developing heart disease within the next 10 years.

3

Symptoms of angina and a heart attack?

Phil Jevon

> **→ Key points**
>
> ◆ If it is the first episode of chest pain, call 999 for an ambulance
> ◆ If previously diagnosed with angina, rest and take GTN as prescribed; if no relief or if concerned, call 999 for an ambulance

---

Introduction

Because it is so important to ensure that, when it is suspected that a patient is having a heart attack, someone immediately calls 999 for an ambulance, it was considered helpful to allocate a chapter in this book aimed specifically at recognising the sympoms of angina and heart attack. These have been discussed in detail elsewhere (see Chapters 5 and 7); a brief outline will be provided here.

The aim of this short chapter is to be able to recognise when chest pain is possibly a heart attack and when it is possibly just angina.

CHD and coronary arteries: related physiology

Partially blocked coronary arteries can hinder blood flow to the myocardium (muscle of the heart). If the heart has to work harder e.g. during exercise, if the muscle doen't receive enough blood and oxygen because of the diseased coronary arteries, chest pain (angina) can result. If the patient rests, the workload of the heart falls and the corresponding blood flow and oxygen demands also falls. The chest pain will usually then resolve, particularly if GTN is administered.

If the coronary artery becomes completely blocked, this causes a heart attack (myocardial infarction). The resultant chest pain will not be relieved by GTN and rest.

Angina: recognising the symptoms

Angina is a symptom of CHD. It can vary from being a mild, uncomfortable feeling in the chest similar to indigestion (mild angina episode) to a severe angina attack causing a feeling of heaviness or tightness, usually in the centre of the chest. Sometimes it is described as a tight vice around the chest. The pain can radiate (spread) to the arms (particularly the left arm), neck, jaw, back or stomach.

Angina is often triggered by physical activity or a stressful or emotional situation e.g. watching an important football match. The symptoms are usually relieved by sitting down and resting and/or taking a GTN spray or tablet.

Heart attack: recognising the symptoms

NB If you think you are having a heart attack, dial 999 for immediate medical assistance.

The discomfort or pain associated with a heart attack is similar to that of angina except that it can come on while at rest, is usually more severe and is not relieved by GTN spray or tablets.

Other symptoms that may be associated with a heart attack include:

◆ sweating
◆ light-headedness
◆ nausea and vomiting
◆ breathlessness

NB Some patients who have a heart attack do not experience chest pain.

Women in particular may just get pain in the back, neck and jaw.

4

What are the investigations for angina?

Phil Jevon and Emma Simkiss

> ### → Key points
>
> ◆ Investigations for angina are important to help confirm the correct diagnosis
> ◆ The 12 lead ECG is the most commonly used test
> ◆ Exercise tolerance test, MPI and coronary angiogram are other available tests available to the cardiologist

Introduction

The patient's symptoms of angina can sometimes be very easy to recognise and the cardiologist can confidently make a diagnosis of angina. Investigations can assist in making a diagnosis of CHD and the associated angina.

The aim of this chapter is to describe investigations commonly used for angina.

Routine blood tests

Routine blood tests for angina may include:

Full blood count

A low haemoglobin (HB) or blood count (anaemia) may be the underlying cause of the chest pain.

Cholesterol and triglycerides (lipids) levels

Cholesterol, a fatty substance found in the blood, is mainly manufactured in the body. Although cholesterol is important for the functioning of the body, too much of it can increase the risk of CHS. Cholesterol is transported around the body by lipoproteins, of which there are two types:

◆ *LDL* (low-density lipoprotein): too much of this is harmful and can increase the risk of CHD

◆ *HDL* (high-density lipoprotein): is a protective type of cholesterol

Triglycerides are fatty substances found in the blood. Being overwieght, a diet high in fatty and sugary foods and a high intake of alcohol will increase triglyceride levels in the blood. Elevated triglyceride levels in the blood are associated with increased risk of CHD.

Cardiac enzymes

In some patients, it is difficult to distinguish whether the patient has had an episode of angina or a heart attack. The cardiologist will usually then take a blood sample to measure the levels of cardiac enzymes. Cardiac enzymes are released by damaged heart cells into the blood stream when the patient has suffered a heart attack.

The levels of two types of cardiac enzymes are usually measured:

◆ *Troponin (T)*: released into the blood stream 2–6 hours after a heart attack; with levels peaking at about 24 hours

◆ *Kinase (K)*: released into the blood stream 4–6 hours after a heart attack, with levels peaking at about 24 hours

The 12 lead ECG

The 12 lead ECG is an essential diagnostic tool in the management of heart disease, in particular angina and heart attack.

Definitions

An electrocardiograph is a machine that records the waveforms generated by the heart's electrical activity in its conduction system (see Chapter 1). The electrocardiogram (ECG) (Fig. 4.1) is a record or display of a person's heart-beat produced by an electrocardiograph. The term ECG is commonly used to describe both the electrocardiograph and electrocardiogram.

What the 12 lead ECG records

The heart generates electrical forces, which travel in multiple directions simul- taneously. If the flow of current is recorded in several planes, a comprehensive view of this electrical activity can be obtained.

Although it is called a 12 lead ECG, only ten ECG cables are actually con- nected to the patient: four to the limbs and six to the chest. Attaching these ten cables enables the ECG machine to record the electrical activity of the heart from 12 different angles.

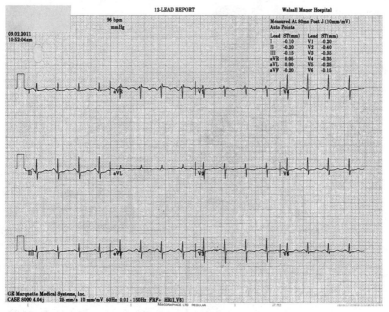

Figure 4.1 Electrocardiogram (ECG)

Reasons for recording a 12 lead ECG

The most common reason for recording a 12 lead ECG is chest pain i.e. the clinician suspects a possible cardiac event such as angina or heart attack. There are, however, lots of other reasons for recording an ECG including history of collapse, palpitations or sometimes prior to a general anaesthetic.

Procedure

It is important to be relaxed and to breathe normally during the recording of a 12 lead ECG. If the patient is shivering or moving, then the ECG trace recorded may be distorted and difficult to interpret. The patient is usually asked to lie down on an examination couch or bed in a semi-recumbent position e.g. resting against a pillow at an angle of 45 degrees with the head well supported. The arms are placed at the sides of the patient with the inner aspects of the wrists close to, but not touching, the patient's waist (Fig. 4.2). The patient's chest will need to be exposed and if necessary the skin is prepared e.g. if the patient has a very hairy chest, it may be necessary to shave the areas where the chest electrodes are going to be attached. Six electrodes are carefully placed on the chest, and four on the inner wrists and inner parts of both lower legs just above the ankles. The ECG cables are then connected to the ten electrodes. Sometimes different electrode positions are used.

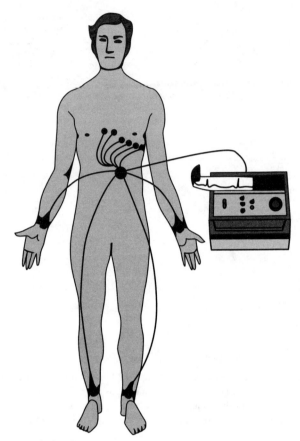

Figure 4.2 ECG (Taken from Heart Disease: The Facts)

What the standard 12 lead ECG records

The standard 12 lead ECG records the electrical activity of the heart from 12 different viewpoints or leads ('leads' are viewpoints of the heart's electrical activity, they do not refer to the cables or wires which connect the patient to the monitor or ECG machine) by attaching 10 leads to the patient's limbs and chest.

Electrical current flows between two poles, a positive one and a negative one. An upward deflection will be recorded on the ECG when the current is flowing towards the positive pole; whereas a downward deflection will be recorded if the current is flowing away from the positive pole. This can clearly be seen in the ECG in Fig. 4.1 where the deflections of the ECG vary from lead to lead.

Interpretation of the 12 lead ECG

The 12 lead ECG can provide a lot of invaluable and helpful information relating to heart disease. In respect of angina and heart attack, key abnormal differences to the normal ECG trace can usually be seen.

Although a normal ECG is obviously a good sign, it must be stressed that a normal ECG does not necessarily mean that the patient does not have CHD e.g. some patients with a history of chest pain while exercising have a normal ECG at rest but, during an exercise ECG test (see below), develop an abnormal ECG with changes indicating the presence of CHD.

Exercise tolerance test

An exercise tolerance test (ETT) involves continous monitoring of the ECG while the patient exercises, usually on an exercise bike or a treadmill. The level of exercise is gradually increased i.e. the workload of the heart is gradually increased.

An ETT can be used to measure how much exercise the patient's heart is able to tolerate before the symptoms of angina are triggered. This information is useful for assessing the likely severity of your angina. Exercise tolerance testing (ETT) is an important diagnostic and prognostic test to assess a patient with either known or suspected CHD.

The mode of exercise can be walking on a treadmill or riding a bicycle. The patient will be connected up to a 12 lead ECG and automated blood pressure monitor. The aim of the exercise is for the patient to achieve at least 85% of their maximum predicted heart rate which is calculated as follows:

- Men: 220 minus the age of the patient
- Women: 210 minus the age of the patient

The cardiologist will advise that beta blocker medications should be discontinued the day before and on the day of the test and digoxin should be stopped one week before testing. Patients are advised to wear loose, comfortable clothing.

ETT will typically take about half an hour, with the exercise regime gradually increasing over a 21 minute period. However, the ETT may be stopped at any time. The most common reason for stopping an exercise test is fatigue and breathlessness as a result of the unaccustomed exercise. If the patient develops chest pain or irregularities on the ECG are other reasons to terminate the test.

Complications

Serious complications e.g. heart attack can very rarely occur (incidence of 1:10,000 tests (0.01%)). As cardiac arrest can occur (incidence 1 in 5000), resuscitation facilities including a defibrillator will be immediately available.

Myocardial perfusion imaging (MPI)

Although dynamic exercise testing (e.g. on a treadmill) is the stress technique of choice, it is not always appropriate, feasible or indeed safe for patients e.g. inability or poor motivation to perform dynamic exercise or recent exercise ECG with inadequate exercise.

MPI is recommended by The National Institute for Clinical Excellence (NICE) as the initial diagnostic tool for people with suspected CHD for whom dynamic exercise testing (see above) poses particular problems: women, left bundle branch block on the ECG, diabetics and those unable to do treadmill tests. It is a noninvasive diagnostic tool that can then provide valuable information on coronary blood flow both at rest and during stress. It is highly likely that a patient with suspected or indeed confirmed angina will be referred for MPI.

MPI is undertaken in the Nuclear Medicine Department. Nuclear Medicine uses radioactive isotopes in the diagnosis and treatment of disease. In diagnosis, radioactive substances are administered to patients and the radiation emitted is detected using a Gamma Camera (Fig. 4.3).

The foetal dose of radiation is relatively high in MPI imaging. It is therefore important to ensure that the patient is not pregnant: ladies of child bearing age should comply with the 28 day rule (that they are within 28 days of the first day of their last period) and sign a declaration to show they understand a radiation dose will be administered and they are confident they are not pregnant. It is also advisable that prolonged contact between the patient and small children/pregnant ladies is avoided for 24 hours.

Indications for a MPI include:

◆ Assessing the presence and degree of coronary artery obstruction in patients with suspected CHD

◆ Assisting the management of patients with known CHD e.g. determining the likelihood of future coronary events, guiding strategies of myocardial revascularization (opening-up of the coronary arteries)

Coronary circulation and exercise: related anatomy and physiology

During exercise, normal coronary arteries will dilate, ensuring the blood flow to the muscle of the heart (myocardium) increases to meet its demands. Coronary arteries with >70% stenosis (narrowing) can usually maintain

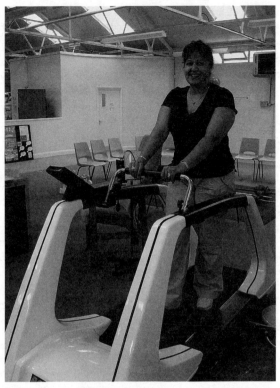

Figure 4.3 Exercising on a treadmill

Reproduced with kind permission of Walsall Cardiac Rehabilitation Trust (Heart Care) www.heartcare.org.uk

sufficient blood flow to meet the varying oxygen demands of the heart muscle (myocardium).

However, coronary arteries with > 70% stenosis (narrowing) are unable to maintain coronary blood reserve during increased workload of the muscle of the heart. This will result in a relative reduction in coronary blood flow to the affected region of myocardium. These patients may be symptomatic e.g. develop chest pain and/or breathlessness during exercise, but asymptomatic (have no symptoms) at rest.

For details on the anatomy and physiology of the heart, see Chapter 1.

Role of the isotope

Once injected, the isotope (radioactive dye which shows up on an X-ray image) is absorbed by the working myocardium (heart muscle). The isotope will show up very clearly and extensively in areas of the myocardium which have a good blood supply. However, reduced or no absorption of the isotope (called cold spots) will be evident in areas of the myocardium that have a poor or no blood supply.

- Cold spots that appear on both rest and stress images suggest a previous myocardial infarction (heart attack)
- Cold spots that appear on stress but not rest images suggest reversible or exercise induced ischaemia

Adenosine and dobutamine

Myocardial perfusion imaging (MPI) using pharmaceutical stress testing is considered a good alternative. The two types of pharmacological stress tests used are vasodilator stress e.g. adenosine and dobutamine stress.

Adenosine is the most commonly used drug for pharmaceutical stress testing. A naturally occurring product, it increases the blood flow to the myocardium. Side effects can occur including transient facial flush, chest pain, breathlessness, choking sensation and light-headedness. Rarely, bronchospasm (narrowing of the lower airways) can occur resulting in wheezy breathing (this is why it is not administered in asthmatic patients). Fortunately, the above side effects are usually very short-lived (normally lasting only seconds or a few minutes).

As caffeine can block the effect of adenosine, tea and coffee should be avoided 24 hours prior to the test.

The adenosine test typically lasts for 6 minutes (3 minutes of the drug, then the injection of the isotope, and then 3 further minutes of the drug).

Dobutamine is sometimes used, but usually only if there is a contra-indication to adenosine e.g. asthma. It is administered over a 15–20 minute period, with the dose being gradually increased. The aim is to increase the heart rate until it reaches 85% of the maximum predicted heart rate for that patient (see above). Drugs that can block its effect e.g. beta-blockers, should be omitted for 24 hours prior to the test.

Procedure for pharmacological stress test

The procedure for the pharmaceutical stress test (Fig. 4.4) does vary slightly from hospital to hospital. Some key considerations:

- Tea/coffee will need to be omitted for adenosine test (see above) as well as possible certain medications
- Patients are advised to not eat anything for 6 hours prior to the test
- Patients are advised to bring in something 'fatty' to eat e.g. a cheese sandwich or a chocolate bar following the test—this will help to improve the X-rays that are obtained

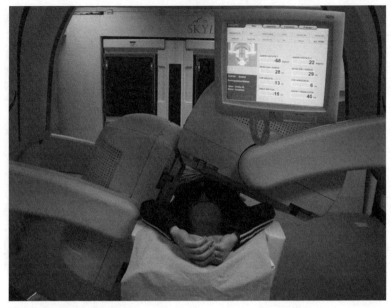

Figure 4.4 Gamma camera

- Patients are weighed before the test—the dose of the drug used is based on the patient's weight

- A cannula will be inserted so that an intravenous infusion of the drug can be administered

- 12 lead ECG monitoring and blood pressure monitoring will be established

- Following the procedure, patients have something fatty to eat (see above) and then return for the scan, typically 30 minutes later. The scan usually takes about 20 minutes.

Scan at rest

A scan will also be performed with the patient at rest. This is usually undertaken on a separate day. The isotope will be administered intravenously.

Coronary angiogram

A coronary angiogram (sometimes called cardiac catheterisation) is a special X-ray test that enables the cardiologist to establish whether CHD is present and the extent to which it is. It can then help determine the most appropriate treatment (if any) for the patient e.g. angioplasty, coronary artery bypass graft

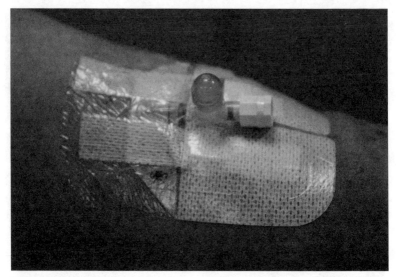

Figure 4.5 Insertion of a Cannula

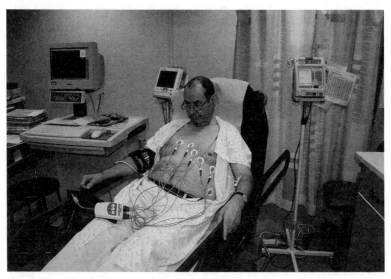

Figure 4.6 Patient being prepared for pharmaceutical stress test

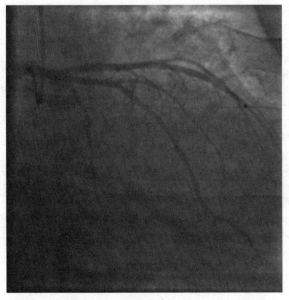

Figure 4.7 Coronary angiogram: X-ray image of the coronary arteries

or medical therapy. A radiopaque (shows up on X-ray) dye is inserted in the coronary arteries and then X-ray images are taken (Fig. 4.4). The procedure is usually undertaken as a day case i.e. it is not usually necessary for the patient to stay in hospital overnight.

Indications

Patients are referred for a coronary angiogram if:

- The diagnosis of angina remains unclear
- The patient's angina symptoms persist despite medical treatment
- There is a high risk that the patient may have a heart attack and coronary artery bypass graft is being considered

Procedure

- The patient is asked to remain nil by mouth for 4 hours prior to the procedure
- The procedure is undertaken in the cardiac catheterisation lab (cath lab)
- The patient removes clothes, dons a gown and lies on a special 'X-ray table'
- A local anaesthetic is injected in the area where the catheter is going to be inserted e.g. groin or arm. This is to numb the area

◆ A catheter is inserted into an artery either in the groin or the arm; the catheter is then advanced using X-ray vision to the coronary arteries. During insertion of the catheter, the patient may feel some slight pressure, but no pain

◆ The radiopaque dye is then inserted through the catheter. The patient usually experiences a brief hot flushing sensation which lasts for approximately twenty seconds. Occasionally the patient feels some chest discomfort when the dye is injected. The patient may feel an urge to urinate

◆ X-rays are then taken which will identify if there are any narrowed areas or blockages in the coronary arteries

◆ Angioplasty and a stent may be performed

◆ Following the test, the catheter is removed and a sterile pad placed over the wound site and direct pressure applied for 15 minutes or even longer to ensure that bleeding does not occur

◆ The patient then rests quietly on a bed, typically for several hours (lying flat if the artery in the groin is used for catheter insertion)

Risks assocated with a coronary angiogram

Although a coronary angiogram is a relatively safe test, complications can very occasionally occur. For example:

◆ Bleeding into the tissues around where the catheter was inserted. Blood collects under the skin (haematoma) which may be uncomfortable and cause bruising.

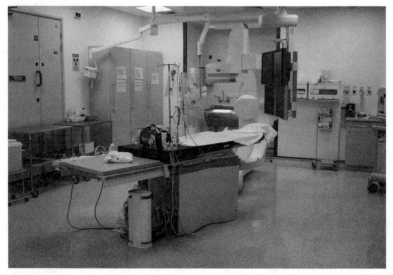

Figure 4.8 A cardiac catheterisation lab

◆ Heart attack, stroke or dying (estimated frequency is 1:1000 patients). The risk of one of these major complications does depend on the patient's overall health and cardiac condition. It must be stressed that the cardiologist would only recommend a coronary angiogram if the benefits outweighed the very small risk.

5

Treatment for angina

Fraz Umar

→ Key points

- Angina is a symptom of CHD
- Lifestyle changes e.g. stopping smoking, reduction in weight may be sufficient to prevent episodes of angina
- Medications e.g. nitrates, can help prevent pain from occurring
- Angioplasty and coronary artery bypass graft surgery may be required

Introduction

Angina is a symptom of CHD. Once the diagnosis of angina is made, the next step is to attempt to 'treat' it. Treatment will vary depending on several factors such as how frequently the symptoms occur and during what level of exertion. This information can be used to assess severity. Treatment can be in the form of drug therapy, angioplasty or surgery along with lifestyle changes which include smoking cessation, weight loss, and dietary changes. Treating precipitating causes of angina can also improve symptoms.

The aim of this chapter is to outline the treatment for angina.

Key treatment options

The actual treatment options considered will obviously depend on the patient. Key treatment options for angina include:

- Smoking cessation
- Diet
- Medications
- Weight loss

◆ Angioplasty

◆ Surgery—coronary artery bypass graft (CABG)

Each will now be discussed in turn.

Smoking cessation

Smoking is a major risk factor for CHD. The stopping of smoking has been shown to reduce the risk of coronary artery disease. Studies have also revealed that stopping smoking is one of the most effective ways of managing CHD. Patients with established CHD on medical therapy, smoking cessation provided added benefit in reducing the risk of having a heart attack. For advice and medical help with quitting please see your GP. There are nicotine replacement products available from local pharmacists. The risk of having a heart attack decreases to the same level as for a non-smoker in about 10–15 years.

Diet

Eating healthy will help prevent your symptoms of angina from getting worse by delaying the narrowing of the coronary arteries. This is best achieved by reducing the amount of fat intake, increasing carbohydrate intake as well as fruit and vegetables. Eating fatty products that contain saturated fats are linked with high cholesterol and therefore aid the development of atheroma. Reducing the amount of red meat and increasing fish and white meat, e.g. chicken, consumed will all help improve your diet.

Weight loss

Losing weight can be difficult but it been has shown to be effective in controlling risk factors which would accelerate CHD such as hypertension and diabetes. The GP can offer you advice on losing weight.

Precipitating causes

Precipitating causes such as low blood count, abnormal irregular heart rate, hyperactive thyroid or severe narrowing of the heart valves could worsen symptoms of angina. Treatment of underlying cause could potentially improve the symptoms or even cure it. Sometimes despite treatment there is no improvement in symptoms. The reason for this could be due to disease of the coronary arteries.

Medications

Treatment with medications can be classified as follows:

◆ Medications that mainly control symptoms i.e. nitrates, calcium channel blockers and potassium channels activators; also fitting into this classification are newly launched medications ivabradine and ranolazine

◆ Medications that improve prognosis by preventing angina and heart attacks i.e. beta-blockers and anti-platelets

◆ Medications that act on precipitating factors of CHD i.e. hypertension and hypercholesterolaemia

Each will now be discussed in turn.

Anti-platelets prevent the sticking of platelets to each other, thus stopping clots forming in the arteries.

Aspirin

Aspirin, a very old drug, reduces the risk of heart attack in patients with CHD by preventing the formation of clots. It is patients who are diagnosed with CHD that benefit the most. In the UK, aspirin 75mg is usually prescribed, though higher doses can be used. Higher doses are associated with increased risk of bleeding.

Common side effects include allergic reaction, indigestion due to inflammation of stomach lining and increased risk of bruising and bleeding including from the intestinal tract.

Clopidogrel

Clopidogrel (Plavix®), a thienopyridoine, also prevents platelets from clotting. It is used as an alternative to aspirin or as an add on therapy especially if an angioplasty with stenting of an artery has been performed. The length of treatment can vary between a month to lifetime. Following stent insertion, clopidogrel should be continued for a minimum of one year. It is usually prescribed as 75mg once daily. It should not be stopped without seeking medical advice first.

Common side effects include rash, bleeding, dizziness, and bruising.

Prasugrel

Another recent addition is Prasugrel (Efient®). This drug has recently been introduced in the UK and is currently only licensed with aspirin for use in patients with acute myocardial infarction. Other indications include the formation of blood clots in a stented artery while being treated with clopidogrel or the patient is diabetic. Prasugrel has been shown to be a more potent anti-platelet agent compared to clopidogrel. Due to higher risk of bleeding in patients older than 75 years and in those who weigh less than 60 kg, with a history of stroke or transient ischemic attack, the recommended dose is half the normal prescription. The current recommended dose is 10mg.

Beta-blockers

Are a group of drugs that are prescribed for various reasons including CHD as well as after a heart attack. In angina and CHD, they reduce the effects of adrenaline and other stress hormones and in doing so slow the heart rate. This in turn has the effect of reducing the workload of the heart and oxygen demand. There are various beta-blockers available and therefore the decision to choose one over the other is more a personal choice of the doctor but also how heart specific the drug should be. Commonly prescribed beta blockers include bisoprolol and atenolol.

Beta-blockers are contraindicated in asthma and bronchitis. Common side effects include general lethargy, nightmares, erectile dysfunction and worsening of peripheral circulation.

Nitrates

Nitrates are medications that release nitric oxide, a smooth muscle relaxant, causing dilatation of coronary arteries with improvement in blood flow. These medications are available in different formats which include tablets, sprays and patches. Long acting preparations are also available for once a day usage.

Most common side effects include headache, lightheadedness and flushing. Nitrates should not be taken with other medications such as Sildenafil (Viagra®).

Potassium channel activators

These drugs have a similar action to nitrates. Nicorandil is used to control symptoms of angina. Initial dose is 10mg twice a day up to 30mg twice a day.

Common side effects are similar to nitrates.

Calcium Channel blockers

Calcium channel blockers lower blood pressure but also have the added effect that they reduce the heart rate and therefore, similar to beta-blockers, help prevent angina. This group of medication is usually used if there an allergy to beta-blockers or if there is history of asthma. There are many different companies producing these tablets and therefore the preparations and dosage differ.

Common side effects include headache and dizziness.

Ivabradine (Procoralan®)

Is a relatively new drug on the market. It has a very different mode of action compared to other anti-anginal medications. It works by reducing the heart rate. As this medication works on different receptors it can be used in patients with asthma and chronic bronchitis. It is usually used as add on therapy if other anti-angina medications have failed to control symptoms. The recommended dose is 5mg twice a day for four weeks. The dose can then be increased to 7.5mg twice a day if tolerated.

Common side effects are related to slowing of the heart rate such as dizziness, low blood pressure and lethargy. Caution is advised if there are existing problems with the heart's conduction system.

Ranolazine (Ranexa®)

Ranolazine is a new drug in the UK for treatment of chronic stable angina. It can be used in conjunction with other groups of anti angina medication such as beta-blockers and calcium channel blockers. The advantages of ranolazine is that it has no effect on heart rate and blood pressure. Therefore it is particularly suitable for patients on maximal anti-angina medications who continue to get angina. Caution is advised when taking other drugs such as digoxin, simvastatin, calcium channel blockers and anti-arrhythmic drugs.

Common side effects include bronchospasm, tiredness, hallucinations, insomnia, erectile dysfunction, fatigue, hypotension, and nightmares.

Cholesterol lowering drugs

Cholesterol lowering drugs called statins do not help in controlling symptoms of angina but they can prevent coronary artery disease from progressing. Commonly used statins include simvastatin and atorvastatin.

Statins reduce total cholesterol including LDL cholesterol. Common side effects include muscle pain, liver injury, and nerve pain called neuropathy. Statins are contraindicated in liver disease.

Other medications used to treat raised cholesterol include fibrates and ezetimibe (Ezetrol®). Ezetemibe reduces cholesterol by decreasing the amount of cholesterol being absorbed from the intestines. It can be added to statins or used on its own. It is prescribed as 10mg once a day. Common side effects include headache, muscle pain, and lethargy.

Angioplasty

Angioplasty is similar to a coronary angiogram, the difference being that in angioplasty the narrowed artery is opened using balloon and stent to improve blood flow and relieve symptoms of angina. Angioplasty is also used in an emergency to treat a heart attack or unstable angina.

The procedure involves inserting a catheter (hollow tube) into an artery in the wrist or groin through which fine hollow tubes are inserted to coronary arteries. X-ray machines that are used to take pictures of the arteries are also used to guide the balloon and stent into position before being inflated to high pressures within the artery. This procedure pushes the atheroma to one side with the stent which is a small metal mesh to keep the atheroma from causing a narrowing again.

There are two types of stents that are currently being used. Bare metal stents and drug eluting stents. The reason for choosing one stent over the other depends on the anatomy, size of the artery, length of the narrowing, and if there is history of diabetes. As a general rule, large arteries with short narrowings are treated with bare metal stents. Routine angioplasty is nowadays performed as a day case procedure and only in rare circumstances requires admission overnight. There is a one in 100 risk of stroke and heart attack, a one in 500 risk of damage to the arteries requiring an emergency bypass operation, and a one in 200 risk of bleeding and bruising from the site of access.

Coronary Artery Bypass Graft

If coronary artery disease has progressed such there are multiple vessels that are occluded or narrowed, coronary artery bypass surgery may be offered. Surgery has been shown to be effective in treating angina as well as improving prognosis. Coronary artery bypass surgery is a common procedure in the UK. It is carried out in specialist cardiothoracic centres.

The number of diseased arteries will dictate how many grafts are needed. Grafts are either veins which are taken from the leg or arms to go around the narrowing. Quite often an artery is also used which is taken from the inside of the chest wall and runs parallel to the breastbone. This artery is called the internal mammary artery. The recovery from heart surgery depends on numerous factors but, in general, a seven to ten day recovery period can be expected. This usually includes a few days in intensive care followed by convalescence on the ward before returning home. Following surgery a full recovery takes approximately 4–6 weeks.

6

Living with angina

Phil Jevon

 Key points

- Despite having a diagnosis of angina, it is still possible to lead a normal life

- Lifestyle changes are usually required, firstly to reduce the risk of worsening the CHD and secondly to reduce the workload of the heart

- It is important to take medications as prescribed; GTN should always be available

- Call 999 if a heart attack is suspected

Introduction

In the UK, many people with angina lead a good quality of life and continue with their normal daily routines and activities. What is important is that, once diagnosed with angina, the patient follows the advice of their doctor or cardiac nurse and takes the necessary steps and makes the recommended lifestyle changes to help ensure a good quality of life and minimise the risk of the CHD worsening.

Although it is not possible to reverse CHD, steps can be taken to help prevent the CHD and angina getting worse e.g. stopping smoking. In addition, it is important to be able to effectively and safely manage episodes of chest pain and recognise when it is more severe and possibly a heart attack.

The aim of this chapter is to understand how to live with angina.

Identification of the risk factors for CHD

It is important to identify the risk factors for CHD, some of which can then be removed or at the very least reduced. The following risk factors for CHD can be addressed (i.e. minimized or removed) thus reducing the risk of a further cardiac event:

- Smoking
- Hypertension (high blood pressure)
- High blood cholesterol
- Physical inactivity
- Overweight
- Diabetes

Smoking cessation

Smoking is major risk factor for CHD; smokers are almost twice as likely to have a heart attack as those who have never smoked. A smoker with diagnosed angina who chooses to continue to smoke therefore runs a very high risk of having a heart attack. Smoking of course also increases the risk of other diseases e.g. lung cancer.

The harmful effects smoking can have on the heart include:

- Damage to the lining of the coronary arteries; this results in fatty material (atheroma) building up in the lining which reduces the size of the lumen (space) for the blood going to the myocardium to pass through. This condition is called atherosclerosis (see Chapter 1)
- Reduction in the oxygen carrying capability of the blood due to the carbon monoxide content of cigarette smoke
- Increased workload of the heart: nicotine in cigarettes acts as a stimulant, adrenaline is produced by the body which increases the heart rate and the force of contraction of the myocardium
- Increases blood pressure: again nicotine in cigarettes acts as a stimulant, adrenaline is produced by the body which increases blood pressure which will increase the workload of the myocardium
- Increased risk of thrombosis (blood clotting)

Passive smoking (being in the same place as another person who is smoking) is also harmful. Research has shown that a non-smoker, who lives with a smoker, has a higher risk of CHD than a person who doesn't.

How to give up smoking

Although giving up smoking is not easy, it is of course achievable. In the UK, 11 million people have successfully given up smoking. However, it can be very difficult to do so. Different strategies have been shown to be successful with different people. The bottom line is that the person must be determined to give up. Sometimes for some people giving up is not too much of a problem, but not re-starting again can be extremely difficult to resist.

Some suggested practical tips to increase the chances of successfully giving up smoking and not re-starting again include:

◆ Make a date to stop smoking and stick to it; telling your partner/spouse and family can be helpful

◆ Try and persuade other smokers in the family to give up at the same time— if they don't the temptation will always be there, as well as the added risk of passive smoking

◆ Get rid of cigarettes, cigarette lighters, matches, ashtrays etc

◆ Discuss a smoking cessation action plan with a suitably qualified professional e.g. GP, practice nurse, etc. Consider nicotine-replacement therapy

◆ Seek advice from other ex-smokers—their advice on how they gave up and, most importantly, how they managed not to start smoking again may be very helpful

◆ Avoid situations which are associated with lighting up a cigarette. Changing the routine may be helpful e.g. go out for a walk

◆ With the money saved from not buying cigarettes, treat yourself and/or your family. This will act as an incentive to continue.

Some people find it helpful to attend a stop smoking clinic or join a stop smoking group. The latter can be particularly helpful—peer pressure to succeed can be very persuasive!

In addition, the following organisations can offer advice on how to stop smoking:

◆ Quit line – telephone 0800 00 22 00

◆ NHS Smoking Helpline – telephone 0800 022 4 332

◆ ASH (Action on Smoking and Health) – telephone 020 7739 5902

Well-balanced diet

Healthy eating is important to help ensure an ideal weight and also to help keep the cholesterol levels in the body within normal limits. It will help to reduce the risk of worsening existing CHD. Although a wide variety of foods can be enjoyed, it is important to eat the rights amounts of each type i.e. a well balanced diet:

◆ *Fruit and vegetables*: approximately one third of the diet

◆ *Starchy foods*: e.g. bread, rice, potatoes and pasta should account for approximately one third of the diet. Wholegrain foods instead of 'white' foods are preferable because they contain more nutrients and fibre and are more filling

◆ *Protein rich foods*: e.g. low-fat milk and dairy foods, lean meat, fish, eggs, beans and other non-dairy sources of protein should account for approximately one third of the diet.

Diet to benefit the heart

Fruit and vegetables

Eating at least five portions of fruit and vegetables each day helps to lower the risk of CHD. The fruit and vegetables can be fresh, frozen or tinned, cooked or raw. It is beneficial to have a variety.

Fish

Eating at least two portions of fish a week is beneficial, particularly if one portion is an oily fish e.g. mackerel, trout or salmon.

Fats

Fats consist of both saturated fats and unsaturated fats (polyunsaturated and monounsaturated). A diet high in saturated fats can lead to a rise in blood cholesterol levels, which increases the risk of CHD. Reducing the amount of foods high in saturated fat (e.g. dairy products) in the diet is therefore very helpful. Small amounts of unsaturated fats e.g. olive, rapeseed and sunflower oils and small amounts of unsalted nuts and seeds is suggested. Eating fish is also very beneficial (see above).

Salt

A high salt intake can lead to hypertension (high blood pressure) which in turn can cause CHD as well as other life-threatening diseases such as stroke and renal (kidney) failure. Therefore, it is very sensible to reduce salt intake. Perhaps use herbs and spices instead of salt to flavour food. A lot of ready-made foods e.g. pre-packed sandwiches, have a high salt content.

Alcohol

High alcohol intake can cause hypertension (high blood pressure) which can cause CHD as well as other life-threatening diseases including stroke and liver failure. In addition, alcohol contains many calories and can contribute to weight gain. The current national recommendations for daily alcohol (units) intake limits are:

- Women: 2–3 units a day
- Men: 3–4 units a day

(A description of units: one small glass of wine or half pint of beer is one unit)

Losing weight

Being overweight can put a great strain on the heart. It can also increase the risk of episodes of angina. In some patients, losing weight at a sensible rate will be a key priority in the lifestyle change management required for angina.

The GP/practice nurse can provide initial advice on what the optimum weight should be and if loss of weight is advisable.

Managing high blood pressure

High blood pressure (hypertension) is a major risk factor for CHD and for having a heart attack. It is therefore important to take steps to try to avoid the development of high blood pressure; if already suffering from high blood pressure, it is important to take steps to help reduce the blood pressure and to take prescribed medications as advised.

Definition of blood pressure

Blood pressure can be defined as the pressure of blood in the circulatory system which is closely related to the force and rate of cardiac contraction and the diameter and elasticity of the arterial walls. There are two readings, a higher systolic reading and a lower diastolic reading:

- *Systolic blood pressure*: peak blood pressure in the artery following ventricular systole (contraction of the heart)
- *Diastolic blood pressure*: level to which the arterial blood pressure falls during ventricular diastole (relaxation of the heart)

Normal blood pressure

The British Heart Foundation advises that a person's blood pressure should be less than 140/85mmHg; however in a patient with CHD and angina the blood pressure should ideally be less than 130/80mmHg.

How high blood pressure affects the heart

Over a period of time high blood pressure will place extra strain on the heart. If untreated, this can lead to the heart gradually becoming enlarged and contracting less effectively. This condition is called heart failure. High blood pressure is a major risk factor for CHD and for having a heart attack.

Factors that can contribute to high blood pressure

Factors that can cause high blood pressure include:

- Insufficient physical activity
- Obesity
- High salt content in the diet
- Drinking too much alcohol
- Not eating enough fruit and vegetables

Lifestyle changes

Making simple lifestyle changes addressing the above risk factors (discussed elsewhere in this chapter) can help reduce the risk of developing high blood pressure and, where there is existing high blood pressure, can help to reduce the blood pressure to an acceptable level.

Importance of monitoring blood pressure

Hypertension (high blood pressure) is a key risk factor for the development of CHD. It is important to regularly monitor the blood pressure e.g. attend well-person clinics which are offered by most GP practices. If suffering from hypertension, it is important to attend appointments with the doctor/nurse on a regular basis so that the blood pressure can be monitored. It is also important to take any blood pressure medications as advised by the doctor.

Diabetes

Diabetes is a major risk factor for CHD. Consistently high blood glucose levels can affect the coronary arteries, making them more susceptible to developing atheroma (fatty deposits in the lining of the artery walls) (see Chapter 1). Concerning the potential CHD risks associated with diabetes, the following is advised:

- *Non-diabetic patient*: cut the risk of developing diabetes by keeping to an ideal weight and undertaking regular physical exercise as advised by medical staff
- *Diabetic patient*: maintain the blood glucose within recommended levels. This will involve ensuring that diabetic medications are taken as prescribed, the appropriate diet is followed and the condition is monitored as recommended by healthcare staff

Exercise

The heart is a muscle. Like other muscles in the body, it needs exercise to keep in shape.

Benefits

There are many benefits of regular exercise including:

- Reducing the risk of CHD
- Improving general well being
- Helping to control weight
- Helping to reduce blood pressure
- Helping to reduce cholesterol
- Improving mental health

Exercise that can benefit the heart

Exercise that can benefit the heart includes:

- Swimming
- Playing an appropriate sport

- Walking
- Gardening
- Climbing stairs

Starting a programme of exercise

> NB Before starting a programme of exercise, patients with angina are advised to consult their GP for advice.

The British Heart Foundation recommends a programme of exercise that aims to build up to at least 30 minutes of moderate physical activity (i.e. breathing more heavily and feeling warmer) on five or more days a week. If this is not realistic initially, the following is suggested:

- Begin with ten minutes of physical activity at least three times a day, starting slowly at a level suitable for the patient
- Gradually increase the time and frequency until 30 minutes feels achievable
- Select a programme that includes enjoyable activities
- Attempt physical activity every day

NB If chest pain develops during physical exercise, stop immediately

Maintaining the momentum for physical exercise

Maintaining the momentum and enthusiasm for physical exercise can be a challenge. It can be helpful to:

- Keep a diary of exercise
- Set realistic goals for exercise routines
- Organise physical activity to fit in with the daily routine
- Undertake physical activity that is enjoyable
- Exercise with a friend or family member
- Use a pedometer to count the number of steps being taken

Chest pain: another episode of angina or a heart attack?

> NB If a person, who has not been diagnosed with CHD, experiences chest pain, call 999 immediately.

The British Heart Foundation has issued the following advice for persons who have already been diagnosed with CHD and have a glyceryl trinitrate (GTN) spray or GTN tablets at hand. Sometimes, these persons may experience chest pain or discomfort which will often be angina which can be managed in the home environment with GTN and rest. However, it may also be a heart attack.

If a person with confirmed CHD experiences any of the following:

◆ A crushing pain, heaviness or tightness in your chest.

◆ A pain in your arm, throat, neck, jaw, back or stomach.

◆ You may also become sweaty, feel light-headed, sick or become short of breath.

The British Heart Foundation recommends:

◆ Stop what you are doing; sit down and rest.

◆ Take your GTN spray/tablets, according to your doctor or nurse's instructions. The pain should ease within a few minutes—if it doesn't, take a second dose.

◆ If the pain does not ease within a few minutes after your second dose, call 999 immediately.

◆ If you're not allergic to aspirin, chew one adult tablet (300mg). If you don't have any aspirin or you are not sure if you're allergic to aspirin, you should rest until the ambulance arrives.

◆ Even if your symptoms don't match the above but you suspect you're having a heart attack, call 999 immediately.

Medications

Once the diagnosis of angina has been made, the GP or cardiologist may prescribe some medications. It is most important that the medications are taken as prescribed. Medications commonly prescribed for angina include:

Nitrates

This class of drugs help to improve the blood flow through to the myocardium (muscle of the heart) by widening the coronary arteries. They can be used to relieve episodes of angina pain and also prevent it. The sub-lingual (under the tongue administration) preparations (see below) act very quickly (within minutes), though unpleasant side effects can occur e.g. a throbbing headache and lightheadedness

Glyceryl trinitrate (GTN) spray: usually one to two activations of the aerosol spray under the tongue; has a longer lifespan than the tablets (typically two years)

Glyceryl trinitrate (GTN) tablets: usually one to two tablets under the tongue; have a short lifespan (once the bottle is opened, it should be replaced after eight weeks).

It is most important to always have GTN at hand, especially if about to undertake a task or exercise that may induce angina (sometimes the GTN tablets are used to prevent a predictable angina attack i.e. it has happened previously.

Some long acting oral nitatres are also commonly prescribed e.g. isosorbide dinitrate.

Beta-blockers

Beta-blockers are a class of medications that help to reduce the workload of the heart (i.e. demand for oxygen, blood and nutrients decreases) by slowing it down and by reducing the blood pressure. They are effective at preventing angina episodes. Bisoprolol is a commonly prescribed beta-blocker.

Calcium channel blockers

Calcium channel blockers can be used to help prevent episodes of angina. Nifedipine is a commonly prescribed calcium channel blocker for angina, often with a beta-blocker.

Statins

Statins help to reduce the cholesterol. They will usually be prescribed if a person has a raised blood cholesterol level.

7

Treatment of a heart attack

Phil Jevon

 Key points

- Chest pain may indicate a cardiac event such as a heart attack
- Calling 999 for an ambulance at an early stage is paramount
- Chewing aspirin 300mg (if not allergic to aspirin) prior to the arrival of the ambulance service is recommended
- In-hospital treatment of a heart attack includes pain relief, reperfusion therapy and cardiac rehabilitation

Acute coronary syndrome

Coronary means related to the coronary arteries and syndrome means a group of concurrent symptoms of disease. Acute coronary syndrome (ACS) is a commonly used umbrella term when a patient has persistent chest pain or discomfort which appears to be originating from the heart. It can sometimes be difficult for medical staff to determine whether the patient is having a heart attack or an episode of unstable angina.

Difference between angina and unstable angina

Stable angina can be defined as predicable chest pain i.e. it occurs following a certain amount of exercise or stress and is relieved by rest and medications e.g. GTN.

Unstable angina, on the other hand, is when the chest pain occurs for the first time or when previous stable angina (see above) occurs but is worse than normal and/or its characteristics have changed e.g. not relieved by GTN or following a certain amount of exercise that previously has not resulted in chest pain. Unstable angina may suddenly occur leaving the patient feeling very unwell. It is sometimes very difficult to distinguish between unstable angina and a heart attack.

Definition of a heart attack

A heart attack (sometimes called a coronary or coronary thrombosis) is where one of the coronary arteries providing blood to the muscle of the heart becomes blocked e.g. by a blood clot. The area of the heart muscle that receives blood via this blocked artery can be starved of oxygen and subsequently die. The medical term for a heart attack is acute coronary syndrome (the traditional term myocardial infarction is also sometimes used).

Risk factors for a heart attack

The risk factors for a heart attack are the same as for CHD which were discussed in detail in Chapter 2. But, as a reminder, it would be helpful to list them here:

◆ Lack of exercise

◆ Hypertension (high blood pressure)

◆ Smoking

◆ Hypercholesterolaemia (high levels of cholesterol in the blood)

◆ Obesity

◆ Family history of CHD

◆ Diabetes

Heart attack and cardiac arrest

When a person has a heart attack, there is a significant risk of cardiac arrest and sudden cardiac death in the immediate period following the event. The most common cause of this is an abnormal cardiac rhythm called ventricular fibrillation. Instead of the electrical impulses in the conduction system being conducted in a normal and organised way resulting in cardiac contraction and blood flow around the body (see Chapter 1), there is complete electrical chaos in the heart.

Ventricular fibrillation results in the heart quivering or fibrillating instead of contracting normally. Ventricular fibrillation was first observed back in the 19th century, after a patient had a cardiac arrest in the presence of the attending physician. The physician cut a hole in the patient's chest to look at the heart; in the medical literature he wrote that the heart had the appearance of a 'bag of worms' and was not contracting in the normal manner.

Ventricular fibrillation can normally be easily treated by defibrillation. However, for defibrillation to be successful, it needs to be delivered as quickly as possibly following the onset of ventricular fibrillation i.e. within the first few minutes. If ventricular fibrillation occurs while the patient is in the back of an ambulance on the way to hospital or in hospital itself, then immediate defibrillation is possible which is usually successful. However, if ventricular fibrillation occurs outside the healthcare environment then chances of the patient surviving are vastly reduced—prompt CPR and prompt arrival of a defibrillator are crucial.

The significant risk of cardiac arrest is one of the reasons why it is so important to call 999 for an ambulance if it is suspected that a person is having a heart attack. It is therefore very important to be able to recognise the signs and symptoms of a heart attack.

Signs and symptoms of a heart attack

The symptoms of a heart attack can vary from person to person. Classical signs and symptoms include:

◆ Severe central chest pain, often described as a heaviness or tightness in the chest. The pain can radiate to the arms (particularly left arm), neck, jaw, back or stomach.

◆ Nausea

◆ Breathlessness

◆ Sweating

◆ Pallor (pale skin)

◆ Cold and clammy skin

Some patients (women in particular) may only experience pain in the neck, jaw, arms or stomach. Sometimes it is difficult to distinguish between 'chest pain' and indigestion. Sometimes, patients experience very little discomfort (referred to as a silent heart attack) and may not even seek medical advice.

When to call 999 for an ambulance

'Chest pain is your body saying call 999' (British Heart Foundation)

If it is suspected that a person is having a heart attack dial 999 for an ambulance. This is the national recommendation. Patients suffering a heart attack need to get to hospital as soon as possible because:

◆ There is a significant risk of cardiac arrest

◆ Treatments are available that can significantly improve prognosis and post-event quality of life

What to do while waiting for the ambulance

While waiting for the ambulance:

◆ Ask the patient to adopt a comfortable position e.g. sitting down or even lying down if he is feeling light headed

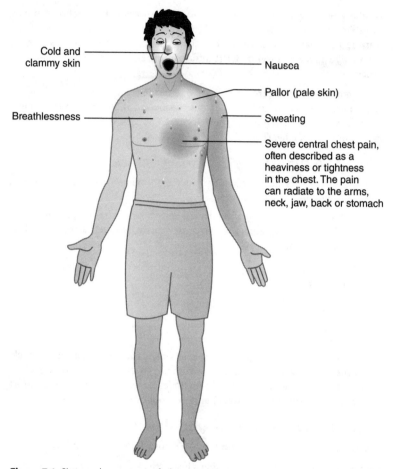

Cold and clammy skin

Nausea

Pallor (pale skin)

Breathlessness

Sweating

Severe central chest pain, often described as a heaviness or tightness in the chest. The pain can radiate to the arms, neck, jaw, back or stomach

Figure 7.1 Signs and symptoms of a heart attack

◆ Ensure there is a 'sick bowl' or similar receptacle at hand as the patient may vomit

◆ If the patient is not allergic to aspirin, offer him aspirin 300mg to be taken orally—ask him to chew it or alternatively, crush it between two teaspoons (suggestion) and then offer it to him. Aspirin is recommended for its anti-blood clotting effect not its analgesic effect. It is important to remember to inform the ambulance service when they arrive that the patient has taken aspirin

◆ If the patient has GTN spray (or tablets) (see Chapter 6) at hand, offer this to him. These should be taken as prescribed by his doctor

◆ Remain with the patient. It is a very frightening time for them—having a loved one near him will be both comforting and reassuring. It is also important to stay with the patient in case he has a cardiac arrest—cardiopulmonary resuscitation will need to be started

◆ Ask another person to look out for the ambulance service. This is very helpful as it can speed up their arrival.

When the ambulance service arrives

Usually an ambulance will be sent to a patient with chest pain (in some remote areas an air ambulance will be sent). However, prior to the arrival of the ambulance, a first responder e.g. paramedic on a motorcycle may be dispatched.

◆ Prior to transfer to hospital, the ambulance service will usually undertake the following:

◆ Administer oxygen via a face mask. Some ambulance services may administer entonox (a mixture of oxygen and nitrous oxide) which can relieve some of the chest pain

◆ Attach pulse oximetry monitoring—a little pleth that is attached to a finger which monitors the oxygen levels in the blood.

◆ Connect ECG monitoring—three sticky electrodes are attached to the chest. ECG cables are then hooked up to these electrodes. The ECG rhythm of the heart can then be closely monitored

◆ Insert a cannula (needle) into a vein. This will allow the delivery of emergency drugs straight into the circulation if they are required

◆ Administer aspirin 300mg (if the patient is not allergic to aspirin and has not already taken it)

◆ Administer GTN spray (or tablet) under the tongue to help relieve some of the pain

Some ambulance services will record a 12 lead ECG and may start thrombolylic therapy (see later in the chapter).

Transfer to hospital

The patient will be transferred to hospital as quickly as possible (via a blue light). Depending on the situation and local facilities, the patient may be transferred to the local A & E department or to the nearest hospital with a cardiac centre. If the latter is the case, then it is possible that the patient will bypass a local hospital.

During transfer, the patient will be continually monitored (ECG and oxygen levels in the blood). A paramedic will be with the patient. Some ambulance services may allow a close relative to travel in the back of the ambulance.

Arrival at the hospital: initial treatment and management priorities

When the patient first arrives at the hospital, he will be taken to where he can be properly assessed by a senior clinician e.g. cardiologist. Initial priorities usually include:

◆ Transferring the patient from the ambulance stretcher to a bed, couch or trolley depending on the locality e.g. in A & E it is likely to be a trolley, in the coronary care unit it will usually be a bed. Unless the patient is feeling light-headed (may suggest a low blood pressure), he will usually be nursed in a semi-recumbent position (lying at an angle of about 45 degrees supported by pillows). Not only is this usually a comfortable position, it is also helpful when recording a 12 lead ECG.

◆ Administering oxygen (guided by the pulse oximeter's measurement of the oxygen levels in the blood). It may not be necessary to administer oxygen.

◆ Inserting a cannula into a peripheral vein e.g. back of the hand or in the fold of the elbow (if not already done by the ambulance service). After taking a blood sample, the cannula will be flushed with a small amount of fluid usually normal saline, to help ensure that it remains patent.

◆ Relieving the chest pain. Obviously, for the patient's comfort, It is very important to adequately relieve the chest pain. It is also important to relieve it because the pain can increase the patient's stress and subsequently the workload of the heart (this needs to be avoided). A strong pain killer such as an opiate e.g. morphine is usually administered through the cannula (see above) straight into the blood stream. It is also standard practice to administer an anti-emetic e.g. cyclizine, because a side effect of morphine is nausea and a patient having a heart attack is also usually nauseous.

◆ Commencing ECG monitoring—particularly so that the nurses and doctors can closely monitor the rhythm of the heart. If ventricular fibrillation (see above) occurs, the ECG monitor will help confirm prompt and correct diagnosis, thus facilitating prompt defibrillation.

◆ Recording a 12 lead ECG to detect any changes which will suggest possible heart attack or unstable angina (Fig. 7.2). The 12 lead ECG will be repeated, possibly several times.

◆ Taking a detailed clinical history. The clinician wanting to establish firstly whether it is likely to be a cardiac event and secondly, if it is, whether it is likely to be a heart attack or unstable angina. In some patients it is very easy to make the correct diagnosis, in others it can be very difficult.

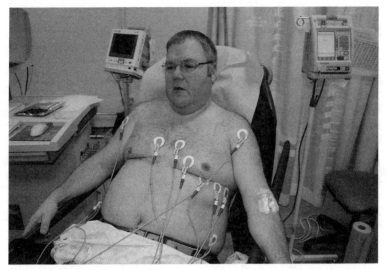

Figure 7.2 Recording a 12 lead ECG

- Taking blood samples e.g. troponin (see below) to establish whether any of the heart has been damaged.
- Ordering a chest X-ray to check the heart and lungs.

Making a diagnosis

The clinician can make a provisional diagnosis of a heart attack based on the clinical history; the diagnosis of heart attack can be confirmed by specific changes on the 12 lead ECG and the results of blood tests:

- Clinical history: not only the clinical signs of a heart attack but also when it is likely it happened. This will affect what treatment is indicated.

- Changes on a 12 lead ECG. The clinician may be able to establish whether a blood clot has caused the abrupt interruption of blood supply to an area of myocardium (muscle of the heart) i.e. a coronary artery is completely blocked—a heart attack. On the ECG, this usually manifests itself initially as ST segment elevation. If a blood clot has only partially blocked a coronary artery this may also be apparent on the ECG e.g. ST segment depression. This could indicate unstable angina, but not a heart attack.

- Blood tests: measuring troponin and cardiac enzymes levels in the bloodstream. Raised levels indicates a heart attack; the extent of the rise indicates the severity/extent of the damage to the myocardium (muscle of the heart).

Troponin

Most hospitals will measure troponin levels in the blood if a heart attack is suspected. Troponins are proteins found in heart muscle and are not normally present in the blood.

They are leaked into the blood if the heart is damaged such as following a heart attack. However, because it can take up to 12 hours after the event for them to be detected, an initial negative troponin does not mean that the patient has not had a heart attack. A repeat troponin will be requested. Some hospitals will only measure troponin levels and not cardiac enzymes.

Cardiac enzymes

Cardiac enzymes e.g. CK and CKMB assist chemical actions in the myocardial muscle cells. If the patient has a heart attack, these enzymes are released into the blood. Elevated levels in the blood (low levels are a normal finding) indicates damage to the myocardium (muscle of the heart). However, it can take between 12 and 24 hours for a significant elevation of these enzymes to be recorded.

Reperfusion therapy

The key treatment strategy for an acute heart attack is reperfusion therapy i.e. opening up the blocked coronary artery. This can be achieved by angioplasty (preferable) and/or thrombolysis.

Reperfusion therapy needs to be undertaken as soon as possible after a heart attack. The earlier it is done, the more myocardium that can be salvaged and the less myocardium that is damaged. This is one of the reasons why it is so important to call 999 for an ambulance if a person develops chest pain.

Thrombolysis

Thrombolysis literally means the breaking down of a blood clot. The administration of a thrombolytic drug e.g. streptokinase, into the blood stream can help to dissolve the blood clot that is blocking the coronary artery, thus helping to restore blood flow through that particular coronary artery to the muscle it supplies.

In some parts of the UK, thrombolysis is started in the pre-hospital phase of a heart attack. Patients who receive thrombolysis, usually have to remain in hospital for several days in order for the cardiologist to monitor their progress. They should also be given a card indicating that they have had the treatment and also the specific drug that was administered (the drug should not be repeated again because there is a risk of a severe allergic reaction). If the patient has another heart attack and thrombolysis is indicated a different drug will be administered.

Coronary angioplasty with stent

Coronary angioplasty with stent is becoming increasingly the treatment of choice for reperfusion therapy. When used to open up the narrowed coronary artery in this situation, it is referred to as primary angioplasty (the medical terminology: percutaneous primary intervention or PCI).

The procedure for primary angioplasty is the same as for coronary angioplasty which is undertaken as a planned procedure and has been described in detail in Chapter 4. Patients can sometimes be discharged from hospital after only a few days.

Medications

A combination of medications will usually be prescribed to help reduce the chances of a blood clot from forming in and blocking a coronary artery, to ease the chest pain and to reduce the likelihood of on-going damage to the myocardium (muscle of the heart). Medications commonly prescribed include:

♦ Heparin: an anticoagulant that is administered via an injection in the skin. It helps to stop the blood from clotting

♦ Aspirin

♦ Clopidogrel

♦ Glycoprotein IIb/IIIa inhibitor

♦ Nitrates

♦ Beta-blocker

♦ ACE inhibitors.

Further tests and investigations

During the period in hospital, further tests and investigations will be carried out including repeat blood tests (troponin and cardiac enzymes), repeat 12 lead ECGs to monitor the recovery of the myocardium (muscle of the heart). While on the coronary care unit or acute cardiac ward, the patient will usually be on continuous ECG monitoring to detect any abnormalities in the rhythm of the heart. This is most likely to occur during the acute phase of a heart attack.

Tests will also be carried out to assess the pumping action of the heart e.g. chest X-ray and echocardiogram. Sometimes following a heart attack the damage to the myocardial muscle can result in the pumping action being compromised. This is referred to as heart failure.

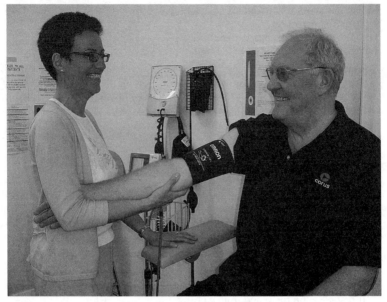

Figure 7.3 A patient having their blood pressure checked

Reproduced with kind permission of Walsall Cardiac Rehabilitation Trust (Heart Care)
www.heartcare.org.uk

Anxiety following a heart attack

Patients who have a heart attack frequently say that it is a very frightening experience. This is made worse by being in a coronary care unit (or similar) with the ECG monitors and other unfamiliar high-tech equipment. Seeing other ill patients can also compound the anxiety.

Even when over the initial acute phase, anxiety can still be a problem. For example, being transferred from a coronary care unit where patients are closely monitored to a general ward where they will not be as closely monitored.

Anxiety can also occur on discharge from hospital, particularly as doctors and nurses are now no longer immediately at hand. To help reduce anxiety, healthcare staff will try to reassure the patient. Cardiac rehabilitation will also help to reduce the anxiety.

Cardiac rehabilitation programme

Patients who have had a heart attack should ideally attend a cardiac rehabilitation programme. Cardiac rehabilitation (sometimes referred to as cardiac rehab) has become an increasingly important aspect of care for cardiac patients, particularly those suffering from a heart attack. It has changed from being perceived as an occasional add-on to care, to becoming an expected and integral part of the care pathway for the treatment and on-going care of a patient following a heart attack. It includes a programme of education and exercise sessions with the purpose of assisting patients to improve their lifestyle and the health of their heart in the hope of reducing the risk of dying from a cardiac event and reducing some of the risk factors for CHD. Cardiac rehabilitation starts while the patient is in hospital.

8

Cardiac rehabilitation: recovering from a heart attack

Phil Jevon

> ## ⮕ Key points
>
> ◆ Cardiac rehabilitation is a programme of education and exercise sessions to improve lifestyle and reduce the risk of a further cardiac event
>
> ◆ All patients who have a heart attack should be invited to join a cardiac rehabilitation programme (where appropriate)
>
> ◆ Wherever possible, the patient's partner/spouse should be actively included/involved in cardiac rehabilitation

Introduction

Cardiac rehabilitation (sometimes referred to as cardiac rehab) over recent years has become an increasingly important aspect of care for cardiac patients, particularly those suffering from angina or following a heart attack (myocardial infarction). Featuring prominently in the Government's National Service Framework (NSF) for Coronary Heart Disease, cardiac rehabilitation has changed from being perceived as an occasional add-on to care, to becoming an expected and integral part of the care package.

Cardiac rehabilitation is a programme of education and exercise sessions with the purpose of assisting patients with certain heart conditions to improve their lifestyle and their heart health. Although not compulsory, it has been shown to reduce the risk of dying from a cardiac event and can reduce the some of the risk factors for CHD.

In this chapter, cardiac rehabilitation following a heart attack will be discussed.

Definition of cardiac rehabilitation

A simple definition of cardiac rehabilitation (or cardiac rehab) is the provision of help and support to a person following a cardiac event cardiac event such as a heart attack.

A more complex definition of cardiac rehabilitation has been provided by the World Health Organisation (WHO):

'… the sum of activities required to influence favourably the underlying cause of the disease, as well as the best possible physical, mental and social conditions, so that they may, by their own efforts preserve or resume when lost, as normal a place as possible in the community. Rehabilitation cannot be regarded as an isolated form of therapy but must be integrated with the whole treatment of which it forms only one facet.'

NSF for Coronary Heart Disease

The Government's National Service Framework (NSF) for Coronary Heart Disease states that UK hospitals should have procedures in place to ensure that those admitted to hospital suffering from coronary heart disease are invited to participate in a multi-disciplinary programme of cardiac rehabilitation. The aim of the programme will be to reduce their risk of subsequent cardiac problems and to promote their return to a full and normal life.

Patients should therefore be able to access adequate cardiac rehabilitation if they are admitted to hospital with a cardiac event. Unfortunately, this is not always the case. The provision of adequate cardiac rehabilitation is subject to the so-called postcode lottery. In addition, in many areas of the UK, patients have to wait for several weeks before they can access cardiac rehabilitation, thus delaying their return to a normal life.

There are also inequalities relating to patients' access to cardiac rehabilitation. For example:

♦ Over 30% of people with CHD are women, yet only 15% of people using cardiac rehabilitation services are women

♦ Ethnic minorities, the elderly and patients with very severe CHD are also under-represented among those who use cardiac rehabilitation services.

Purpose of cardiac rehabilitation

The purpose of cardiac rehabilitation is to help facilitate recovery and to reduce the likelihood of a future cardiac event (often called secondary prevention). Cardiac rehabilitation is an on-going and is generally defined as a process of four phases, which start soon after diagnosis (usually in hospital) and continued through to long term maintenance.

Benefits of cardiac rehabilitation

There is good evidence suggesting that comprehensive cardiac rehabilitation is very beneficial. This is particularly the case when it is individualised and the patient receives help, education and advice relating to lifestyle modification, as well as psychological support, and exercise training. It has been estimated that cardiac rehabilitation may reduce mortality by as much as 20% to 25% over a three year period.

Addressing risk factors for CHD

The following risk factors for CHD can be addressed (i.e. minimized or removed) through cardiac rehabilitation, thus reducing the risk of a further cardiac event:

♦ Smoking
♦ Hypertension (high blood pressure)
♦ High blood cholesterol
♦ Physical inactivity
♦ Overweight
♦ Diabetes

Indications for cardiac rehabilitation

In this chapter cardiac rehabilitation for patients who have had a heart attack is being discussed. However, cardiac rehabilitation can be very beneficial in a number of cardiac conditions including:

♦ Angina
♦ Coronary angioplasty
♦ Cardiac surgery e.g. coronary artery bypass graft surgery
♦ Implantable cardioverter defibrillator (ICD) fitted
♦ Stable heart failure
♦ Cardiomyopathy
♦ Congenital heart disease.

The cardiac rehabilitation team

The cardiac rehabilitation team is usually multi-professional and will include some or all of the following:

♦ *Cardiologist*: lead clinician in charge of the patient's care
♦ *Cardiac rehabilitation nurse specialist*: lead nurse for cardiac rehabilitation; provides the crucial link between the hospital and the community/cardiac rehabilitation team

- *Physiotherapist*: provides advice and support regarding mobility/exercise
- *Exercise specialist*: provides advice and support regarding exercise at the cardiac rehabilitation centre; helps to formulate individualized exercise routines
- *Dietitian*: provides dietary advice about healthy eating options
- *Psychologist*: provides psychological support when necessary e.g. dealing with depression

Outline of a standard cardiac rehabilitation programme

A standard cardiac rehabilitation programme consists of five stages:

- How the patient can access the programme
- Assessment of the patient for suitability for cardiac rehabilitation
- Development of a patient focused individualized care plan for cardiac rehabilitation
- Participation in the cardiac rehabilitation programme
- Follow-up to the cardiac rehabilitation programme

Phases of cardiac rehabilitation

There are five phases of cardiac rehabilitation:

- Phase I: in-hospital period
- Phase II: early discharge period
- Phase III: formal cardiac rehabilitation programme
- Phase IV: long term maintenance of optimum health

Each will now be described in detail.

Phase 1: in-hospital period

Once the patient's condition is stable the process of cardiac rehabilitation can begin. The rehabilitation process during phase I aims to provide relevant information and adequate reassurance. It will also address a number of issues including;

- Risk factor assessment
- Lifestyle adjustment
- Education and advice
- Mobilisation Plan
- Preparation for discharge
- Follow-up advice
- Medication advice

◆ Sexual advice

◆ What to do for ongoing symptoms

◆ Driving/holiday advice

These issues will normally be dealt with in a structured patient assessment.

Communication between healthcare professionals and patients in hospital and particularly in the acute setting is not always effective. This may be helped by the cardiac rehabilitation nurse seeing the patient with their partner or relative. This also helps to acknowledge the importance of the partner receiving information and advice, to help them to cope with the difficulties surrounding what is perceived to be a life-threatening event.

Education and advice is a continuous process, which should commence in hospital at the point of diagnosis and follow through all the phases of cardiac rehabilitation.

Diet

The role of diet may be important for a number of reasons. These will initially be assessed during the patient interview which will reveal:

◆ Height and weight and calculated Body Mass Index (BMI)

◆ Waist circumference

◆ History of hypertension (high blood pressure)

◆ Cholesterol level

◆ History of diabetes

With this information, the patient will be advised to consider relevant dietary modification. Targets are set on an individual basis for weight/BMI and the relevance of reducing cholesterol and blood pressure emphasised.

The evidence for dietary intervention in reducing mortality from coronary heart disease is variable. However, the basis of the so called Mediterranean diet, including increased fruit and vegetables, monounsaturated oil and oily fish, does appear to reduce vascular risk. Limiting salt intake and controlling calorie intake to reduce weight may help to reduce blood pressure and the risk of other complications. Some patients will have co-existing diabetes, and this will need to be controlled during the acute phase, and if required, referral to a diabetic team.

Lipids

The role of cholesterol and its link with increased risk of CHD has been recognised for a number of years. It has been shown that the administration of a statin e.g. simvastatin, reduces the risk of a further major coronary event and lowers mortality rates. All patients admitted to hospital with suspected heart attack should have a non-fasting cholesterol check. It is important that this is taken within the first 24 hours of the cardiac event, otherwise it may be artificially lowered.

The present guidelines advise reducing total cholesterol to <4.0mmol/L or LDL cholesterol to <2.0mmol/L. If it is above this level, treatment with a statin is recommended. Cholesterol levels should be checked prior to their follow-up appointment so that treatment can be adjusted accordingly. Once control has been established, annual checks can be carried out (birthday check). Although statins are generally well tolerated, patients should have liver function tests prior to treatment and again at twelve months. This is to check that the liver is functioning normally. Patients should also be advised to report unexplained muscular pain because myositis (inflammation of muscle) is a rare, but reversible, side effect. Patients should be advised to avoid grapefruit juice as well.

Mobilisation and activity levels

Following a heart attack, patients follow a mobilisation plan, gently increasing activities day by day. A typical mobilisation plan is detailed in Table 8.1. Although most patients will follow a standard plan of mobilisation, it is important that note is taken of the severity of the heart attack and also any symptoms e.g. breathlessness are carefully monitored. For this reason the mobilisation plan should progress in phases and not days, allowing the patient to be assessed each day, and progressed according to the assessment i.e. the mobilisation plan is individualised.

Table 8.1 Mobilisation Plan

Stage 1	Sit out in chair, walk around bed area
Stage 2	Walk one way to bathroom
Stage 3	Walk both ways to bathroom
Stage 4	Fully mobile around ward
Stage 5	Fully mobile. Manages two flights of stairs

It is important that advice is given regarding the early discharge period. This should include basic advice on developing a daily walking plan. Patients are advised that their heart will continue to heal over the next few weeks and that they should continue to gradually increase their activities. They should be advised not to allow themselves to become over tired and should decrease their activity if they become short of breath, develop palpitations or chest discomfort/pain. Although the emphasis of rehabilitation advice is often to be positive, the importance of reporting chest discomfort/pain, particularly the need to call 999 for persisting chest pain which last for longer than 15 minutes, should be stressed.

Smoking

The role of smoking in CHD has been well established. It accounts for one out of every seven deaths from heart disease (Health Development Agency,

2000). The importance of the impact of smoking in heart disease has been emphasised in the NSF for CHD, which devotes an entire standard to this particular risk factor.

Smoking status should be ascertained during the initial patient assessment. In some cases, the event of the heart attack may act as a sufficient trigger to help the patient to quit. Others may require more intensive support.

Various models have been employed both in terms of primary and secondary prevention, to help people stop smoking. A popular model of change is the one proposed by Prochaska and DiClemente in 1983, which views the change process as a cycle and accepts that different people will be at different stages of change, including:

- Not intending to change (Pre-contemplation),
- Thinking about change (Contemplation),
- Planning for change (Preparation),
- The change in behaviour (Action),
- Continuing the changed behaviour (Maintenance)

The model also accepts the concept of relapse and acknowledges that it is common for individuals to move backwards as well as forwards. The model is thus often depicted as circle or spiral. It also emphasises that, with support, a lapse may not become a relapse, and that it often takes a number of attempts to achieve a sustained change in behaviour.

Most smokers appreciate the risk of their habit and although education is important, it is the support that professionals provide that is likely to help individuals to quit. Brief advice from health professionals can be effective in helping smokers to quit. Cardiac rehabilitation staff have the opportunity to provide advice and encouragement to smokers and arrange for them to be supported throughout their rehabilitation.

Since the publication in 1998 of the government's white paper on tobacco, Smoking Kills, there has been an increase in the amount of services available to help reduce the burden of smoking related diseases. Many areas have developed specialist smoking cessation services to help patients to quit. Cardiac rehabilitation staff liaise closely with these services to help those who require further support. This may include the use of pharmacological agents.

Nicotine Replacement Therapy (NRT), available in six different forms, has been shown to be safe when given to smokers with cardiovascular disease post heart attack patients, during the early rehabilitation phase, the benefits of NRT will have to be balanced against any possible risk. All types of NRT have been shown to be effective in helping smokers quit. They reduce the urge to smoke as well as other withdrawal symptoms. The evidence is strongest for smokers of 10 or more a day. Little evidence exists for lighter smokers.

It is important that support is maintained throughout all stages of the rehabilitation process, and that patients are encouraged to seek further advice or support, if required, in the future. This is important, particularly, if individuals start to smoke again. If support was given in a positive and empathetic manner, it is likely that individuals will be more comfortable to seek further help. It is really important if the spouse is a smoker, then he/she should also stop smoking.

Driving: car or motorcycle driving licence holders

Patients should inform their insurance company and check with their doctor before starting to drive again. Most patients who have had a heart attack are advised that they should not drive for at least four weeks (sometimes this is reduced to one week if they have had successful angioplasty). They do not have to routinely inform the Driver Vehicle Licensing Agency (DVLA).

On return to driving, initially patients are advised to keep their journey times short and assess whether driving provokes any symptoms, which should be reported to their doctor. If experiencing regular symptoms and particularly if driving brings these on, their condition should be reviewed.

Driving: bus, coach and lorry driving licence holders

For those who hold special licences (bus, coach and lorry driving licences) other restrictions apply. These licences will be revoked following a heart attack for at least six weeks and patients should inform the DVLA (by post: DVLA, Swansea SA99 1TU or by telephone: 0300 790 6806). The DVLA's medical questionnaire form '*VOCH1*' will need to be completed; it is available to download from the DVLA's website (www.direct.gov.uk).

Specific criteria have to be met for re-instatement of the driving licence: the patient should be able to complete three stages (9 minutes) of a Bruce protocol or equivalent exercise test without signs of cardiovascular dysfunction e.g. angina, syncope, hypotension, significant ventricular rhythm (heart rhythm) disturbance or electrocardiographic (ECG) signs of ischaemia (poor blood supply to the heart muscle). If these criteria are met the licence will be re-instated on a short term basis (3 years) with evaluation required at intervals not exceeding 3 years.

Resumption of sexual activity

This is an important, yet often neglected, area of cardiac rehabilitation advice. It may be ignored due to embarrassment on the part of the patient, professional or both. Resumption of sexual activity is discussed in educational/advice sessions, as well as being included in advice booklets. Information on this topic has been considered as too vague, with comments such as 'take it easy' being used. Clearly advice needs to be appropriate and suitable for the individual. This can only be given, in some circumstances, if the subject is initiated by the health professional (BACR, 1995).

As with other information, the individual situation has to be assessed, including the severity of the heart attack. It is generally not physical incapacity but psychological disturbance which prevents resumption of normal sexual activity. This psychological disturbance may also be seen in the partner/spouse and it is important, therefore, that the advice is given to the partner as well as the patient.

The vast majority of patients convalescing after a heart attack should be able to cope with the physical demands of their normal sexual activity. The physical demand of sexual activity has been assessed in several studies that have equated the mean maximum heart rate at orgasm as 117 beats per minute, similar to that seen by driving in traffic, climbing two flights of stairs or discussing business on the telephone.

Patients should be advised that they should be able to return to their previous levels of sexual activity unless their condition suggests that this is likely to provoke symptoms of chest pain, palpitations, undue breathlessness or extreme fatigue. Patients should be advised to stop their activity if such symptoms arise and to treat appropriately with GTN. They should also be encouraged to report these symptoms to their doctor/nurse in the same way they would if they experienced symptoms whilst walking.

It is likely that many patients will be able to cope with the physical demand of sexual activity within four to six weeks of their heart attack. This may be assessed by their general levels of activity at the time. It may also be assessed in relation to their progress at a cardiac rehabilitation unit or by exercise testing, which is often an integral part of post heart attack follow up.

If the patient reports difficulties in resumption of sexual activity during their recovery, the health professional should interview the patient and partner, taking a full history. This should include assessment of their physical recovery, symptoms, medications, as some e.g. beta-blocker, may affect sexual performance and history of any previous difficulties. In some cases the problem may extend beyond the MI and may require referral to a sexual counsellor or psychologist (Thompson, 1990).

Going back to work

The majority of patients who have a heart attack can go back to their previous job, though the timing of doing so will depend on the severity of the cardiac event and the type of work undertaken. If work involves light duties, returning to work within six weeks is feasible. However, if the work is heavy and strenuous, returning to work may not be advisable until after a few months.

A sensible approach for some patients is to negotiate with employers to return to work gradually e.g. part time and lighter duties initially, before slowing increasing workload. The GP and cardiac rehabilitation staff will be able to offer advice on this issue.

Phase 2: early discharge period

This phase of cardiac rehabilitation is sometimes neglected, although it is a crucial period for patients in terms of adjustment to change. During the hospital phase the patient and family is helped to deal with the shock of their condition and are given security of the hospital surrounds. This can create feelings of insecurity following discharge.

This early discharge period often reflects the gap between acute hospital care and attendance at a cardiac rehabilitation programme. Many rehabilitation programmes have been structured around exercise, and therefore usually allow patients to gently mobilise at home before attending 4–6 weeks later.

It is important to consider ways in which patients and their family can be helped during this period, which may be associated with increased levels of anxiety. It may also be a period in which the patient starts to consider aspects of the recovery not addressed whilst in hospital.

Hospital rehabilitation staff will often give patients a contact number to be used for advice following discharge. It may also be helpful if the rehabilitation staff make contact with the patient in the early stages after discharge. A home visit may overcome some of difficulties encountered with telephone advice. However, this may be difficult to provide for many patients due to the time and also may prove impractical as an outreach service in certain geographical areas.

Developments over recent years have seen an increase in the number of cardiac nurse specialists liaising between the hospital and the community, whose role is to work with patients in the phase II period. They may also provide support for a longer period for patients who are unable to attend a structured rehabilitation programme. Hospital staff should also liaise with colleagues in primary care. This allows the wider health care team to provide support. It also utilises the knowledge that primary care staff will have of their patients.

Some rehabilitation services use home based rehabilitation packages. The Heart Manual is probably the best known of these. This is a six week programme, initially evaluated in Scotland and now supported by the British Heart Foundation and used in many centres throughout the UK. The initial support is given during the hospital phase and the patient is discharged with an advice manual. The manual provides information relevant to physical and psychological recovery and is supported by two audio cassettes for patient and partner providing further advice and relaxation techniques.

Phase 3: formal cardiac rehabilitation programme

This has generally been called the exercise phase of rehabilitation and typically commences 4–6 weeks following hospital discharge. It is common nowadays for phase III programmes to include other aspects of the rehabilitation process.

Most will include an educational package. It is also common for stress management to be offered, particularly for patients who have heightened levels of anxiety, which may be measured throughout the rehabilitation phases. This is often measured using the Hospital Anxiety Depression (HAD) Scale (Zigmund and Snaith, 1983). The exercise component will often last for 6–12 weeks. Many programmes are hospital based, although the geography and local resources often determine the setting.

Prior to taking part in an exercise programme it is typical for the patient to undergo a risk assessment, including an exercise test. This may be used to highlight patients at risk of further ischaemic episodes but may also be used to set the level of exercise to be prescribed. The exercise undertaken should be relevant to the pre-programme risk assessment.

Programmes will typically have exclusion criteria for some patients:

- Multiple heart attacks
- Poor left ventricular function (poor heart muscle function)
- History of chronic congestive heart failure
- Rest or unstable angina
- Complex cardiac arrhythmias (irregularities of the heart rhythm)
- Left main coronary artery or three vessel athersclerosis on angiography

Exercise programmes may be run on a group or individual basis. Local facilities and personnel will often determine this. The exercise programme will typically consist of; pre-activity assessment, including heart rate and blood pressure checks, warm up phase, including stretching and exercises to prepare the individual for the main exercise component:

- *Conditioning phase*: including either continuous or interval training which usually includes exercises which utilise large muscle groups e.g stepping, walking, static cycling
- *Cool-downing phase*: which may be similar to the warm-up phase and allows the body to recover at a steady rate and thus minimises the risk of hypotension and post exercise heart rhythm disturbances.

Phase 4: long term maintenance of optimum health

This is the maintenance phase and will often include continuation of the exercise programme from phase III. This phase may be seen as continuous and will usually see the patient returning to their normal activities and role in society. It is typically where the patient is handed back to primary care and monitored within a secondary prevention framework. This will include the patient being listed on the primary care CHD register and followed up in a secondary prevention clinic.

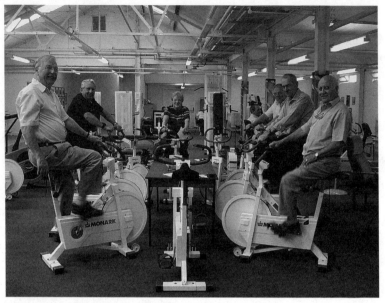

Figure 8.1 Examples of exercise – Static cycling
Reproduced with kind permission of Walsall Cardiac Rehabilitation Trust (Heart Care)
www.heartcare.org.uk

There is a requirement within the NSF for collaboration between secondary and primary care organisations to collect data at one year following recruitment to cardiac rehabilitation. This includes:

- ◆ % taking regular physical activity of at least 30 minutes duration on average 5 times a week

- ◆ % not smoking

- ◆ % whose BMI is below $30kg/m^2$

Strong links between all agencies is required to achieve the targets of the NSF, and this will require systematic pathways of care to be established to streamline services and prevent duplication.

Walsall Heart Care (cardiac rehabilitation service in Walsall, UK) (Fig. 8.1), is a pioneer in cardiac rehabilitation. Since opening in 1981, they have developed a flexible and accessible programme, specially designed to cater for the broadest range of people. Each patient is given a tailor-made exercise programme which is arranged and supervised by the exercise physiology team. The rehabilitation programme is a 13-week course that includes diet and nutrition advice as well as relaxation and stress management therapy for those who need them. Patients must attend two sessions per week.

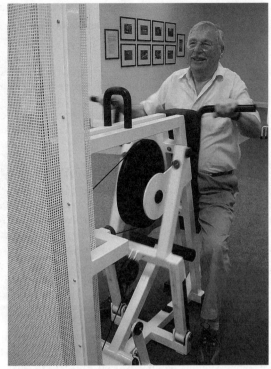

Figure 8.2 Examples of exercise – weight equipment

Reproduced with kind permission of Walsall Cardiac Rehabilitation Trust (Heart Care)
www.heartcare.org.uk

Responsibility of NHS Trusts to provide a cardiac rehabilitation service

NHS Trusts should put in place agreed protocols/systems of care so that, prior to leaving hospital, people admitted to hospital suffering from coronary heart disease have been invited to participate in a multidisciplinary programme of secondary prevention and cardiac rehabilitation. The aim of the programme will be to reduce their risk of subsequent cardiac problems and to promote their return to a full and normal life.

Accessing a local cardiac rehabilitation programme

Patients, who have not already been invited by their hospital onto a cardiac rehabilitation programme, can find out about their nearest cardiac rehabilitation programme by:

◆ Speaking to their GP

◆ Visiting the cardiac rehabilitation website: www.cardiac-rehabilitation.net

◆ Telephoning the British Heart Foundation on 0300 330 3311

Going on holiday

Going on holiday can provide patients an opportunity to unwind and rest. Most patients are fit to fly once they have recovered, assuming their condition is stable. The GP and cardiac rehabilitation team can advise patients whether it is fine to go on holiday and also when it is safe to fly. When booking travel insurance it is usually required to advise the insurance company of the heart attack.

Outpatient appointment: cardiology outpatients

An out-patient appointment with the cardiologist is typically arranged six weeks after being discharged from hospital. The cardiologist will assess how well the patient is recovering and whether changes to medications are required. Some tests e.g. 12 lead ECG will be repeated. Patients often find it helpful to write down questions they wish to ask the cardiologist.

Further reading

British Heart Foundation (2010) G517 *What should I expect from cardiac rehabilitation?*
A guide for heart patients in England British Heart Foundation, London www.bhf.org.uk/publications.

This booklet has been complied by the British Heart Foundation and NHS Improvement Agency for heart patients in response to the Department of Health's new guide (commissioning pack) for the NHS in England relating to cardiac rehabilitation. The purpose of the booklet is to help ensure that a high standard of cardiac rehabilitation services are available for all eligible heart patients.

9

Cardiopulmonary resuscitation

Phil Jevon

> ### ➲ Key points
>
> ◆ Sudden cardiac arrest can complicate CHD
> ◆ Cardiopulmonary resuscitation can be live saving
> ◆ Calling 999, prompt chest compressions and early defibrillation are key initial priorities

Introduction

Each year in the UK about 90,000 people die of a heart attack. One in three people suffering a heart attack die before they even reach hospital. In many of these cases, prompt bystander cardiopulmonary resuscitation (CPR) and prompt defibrillation will significantly increase the chances of the casualty surviving. An understanding of how to perform CPR and to use an automated external defibrillator would therefore be helpful. CPR can be defined as maintaining an open airway and supporting breathing and circulation (sometimes referred to as BLS). Defibrillation is the delivery of an electric shock to the heart.

The aim of this chapter is to understand the principles of cardiopulmonary resuscitation.

Definition of a cardiac arrest

Cardiac arrest literally means that the heart stops. The casualty will collapse, go unconscious, stop breathing and will not have a pulse. There will be no blood circulating around the body. Within a few minutes, unless circulation is restored, irreversible brain damage will occur and death will ensue. Effective CPR will help to maintain circulation and blood flow to the organs in the body, which really need it (vital organs) e.g. the brain and muscle of the heart.

Concept of the chain of survival

Survival from a cardiac arrest relies on a sequence of rapid and effective interventions e.g. calling 999 (or 112) for an ambulance, effective basic life support and prompt defibrillation. These interventions are emphasised nicely in the so-called chain of survival, the concept of which stresses the importance that each time-sensitive intervention must be optimised in order to maximise the chance of survival: a chain is only as strong as its weakest link.

The chain of survival is divided up into four important links:

◆ *Early recognition and call for help to prevent cardiac arrest*: this link stresses the importance of recognizing if a person is at risk of cardiac arrest, calling for help and providing effective treatment to hopefully prevent a cardiac arrest; the majority of people who have a cardiac arrest outside the healthcare setting, have displayed warning symptoms e.g. chest pain prior to collapse. Calling 999 (or 112) for an ambulance is particularly important if a person is complaining of chest pain.

◆ *Early CPR to buy time and early defibrillation to restart the heart*: the two central links in the chain stress the importance of linking CPR and defibrillation as essential components of early resuscitation in an attempt to restore life. While awaiting the arrival of the ambulance service and defibrillator, prompt effective CPR can keep the victim alive. Early defibrillation is particularly important. Many public places such as airports and train stations have a defibrillator. If a defibrillator is available, this should be used as quickly as possible, ideally by a person trained in its use.

◆ *Post resuscitation care to restore quality of life*: the priority initially is to ensure an open airway, adequate breathing and circulation; following a successful resuscitation attempt, placing the victim into the recovery position, can help to prevent the airway from becoming blocked.

Calling 999 (or 112)

The system for calling 999 for the emergency services in the UK has been in operation since 1937. The emergency services include police, fire, ambulance, coastguard, mountain rescue and cave rescue. The European Union has adopted the number 112 for calling the emergency services. In the UK, either 999 or 112 can be called.

999 (or 112) emergency calls are free and can be made from any telephone including a car phone and a mobile phone. If calling from a public call box, no money is needed. If calling from a mobile phone, it is still possible to do so:

◆ Without any credit

◆ If the phone is security locked (the emergency number will override it)

◆ If there is no signal—as long as there is a signal from another mobile phone provider

When the telephone operator answers, he/she will ask which emergency service you require. Tell the operator that you need an ambulance and you will then be connected to the ambulance service (it is important to remember that you call 999 (or 112) for other emergencies as well such as the fire service, police, mountain rescue, coast guard e.g. If there is a fire, you would ask for the fire service).

Once connected to the ambulance service, the ambulance control officer will ask you where you would like the ambulance to come to, the telephone number of the phone you are calling from and details of the emergency. Give accurate details of the address or location where help is needed. If there is a recognizable landmark e.g. famous shop nearby, this information may be helpful. It is important to stay on the line and continue to listen to important advice provided by the ambulance control officer. If at home, ensure family pets are locked away.

Depending on the location and what the emergency is, the Ambulance service may respond with one or more of the following:

◆ Emergency Ambulance

◆ Fast Response Car

◆ Motorcycle

◆ Emergency First Responder

◆ Air Ambulance

The ambulance paramedics and emergency medical technicians are very skilled. To assist them in their work, they will bring along life-saving emergency equipment e.g. oxygen, defibrillator and drugs.

Potential hazards to performing CPR

Even in the emergency situation, it is still important to ensure safety and eliminate, or at least minimise, potential hazards. Potential hazards could include traffic, electricity, gas and infection.

Injury to the rescuer

The actual physical process of performing CPR can result in injury to the rescuer. This of course needs to be ideally avoided or at the very least minimised. Some important considerations:

◆ Assess the situation

◆ Adopt a position close to and directly facing the casualty

◆ Avoid twisting the back

◆ Keep the back in a neutral position

◆ Face the casualty straight on

Initial assessment and sequence of actions in bystander CPR

The initial assessment and sequence of actions in bystander CPR is described in Figs 9.1–9.4. On finding a collapsed, apparently lifeless casualty, ensure it is safe to approach and then check responsiveness.

Unresponsive?: gently shake the casualty's shoulders and ask loudly 'are you all right?' (Fig. 9.1). If the casualty responds, provided there is no further danger, leave him in the position he has been found. If possible, try to establish the likely cause of the collapse; get help or call 999 (or 112) if necessary. If the casualty does not respond, shout out for help.

Shout for help: shout out for help; assistance from other bystanders can be helpful e.g. to call 999 (or 112) for an ambulance, to fetch a defibrillator (AED) or to assist with CPR. Proceed to open the airway.

Open airway: turn the casualty onto his back and open the airway by tilting the head and lifting the chin (Fig. 9.2) (caution if a neck injury suspected—see below) and assess whether he is breathing normally or not.

Not breathing normally?: while maintaining an open airway, assess for no longer than 10 seconds whether the casualty is breathing normally or not:

- Look for movement of the chest
- Listen for breath sounds at the mouth and nose
- Feel for airflow on the cheek

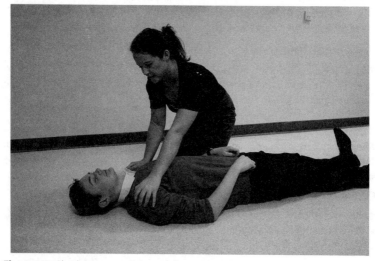

Figure 9.1 Check response: shake and shout

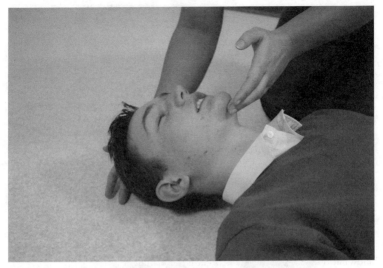

Figure 9.2 Open the airway: head tilt/chin lift

During the first few minutes following a cardiac arrest, the casualty may be hardly breathing or taking infrequent noisy gasps. This is not, and should not be confused with, normal breathing.

If the casualty is not breathing normally, proceed to calling 999 (or 112) for an ambulance.

Call 999: If the casualty is not breathing normally, ask someone to call 999 (or 112) for an ambulance and to fetch a defibrillator if one is available. If alone, call 999 (or 112) from mobile telephone. Only leave the casualty to call for help if there is no other option of doing so. Proceed to 30 chest compressions.

30 chest compressions: deliver 30 chest compressions at a rate of 100–120 per minute (Fig. 9.3). After 30 compressions, proceed to rescue breaths.

2 rescue breaths, 30 compressions: deliver 2 rescue breaths, followed by 30 chest compressions. If not trained to, or unwilling to, deliver rescue breaths, perform chest compressions only at a rate of 100–120 per minute (see compression-only CPR section below).

Continue CPR until help arrives. The rescuer should only stop CPR if:

- Qualified help arrives and takes over
- The casualty begins to breathe normally
- Exhausted

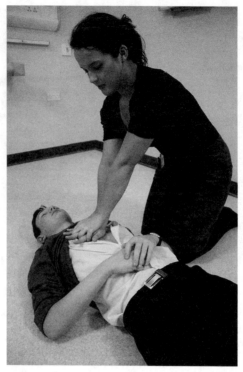

Figure 9.3 Chest compressions

Principles of chest compressions

Chest compressions produce blood flow in the body by increasing pressure in the thoracic (chest) cavity and by directly compressing the heart. The recommended procedure for chest compressions:

1. Ensure the casualty is on his back on a firm flat surface.

2. Kneel at the side of the casualty level with his chest. The knees should be a shoulder-width apart.

3. Place one hand (usually non-dominant one) on the centre of the patient's chest (this is the lower half of the breastbone).

4. Place the other on top of the first hand; do not apply pressure over the end of the breastbone or the upper abdomen (Handley et al., 2005).

5. To avoid applying pressure over the casualty's ribs, interlock and extend the fingers (Fig. 9.4).

6. Position the shoulders directly above the casualty's breastbone, straighten the arms and lock the elbows; ensure the back is not twisted.

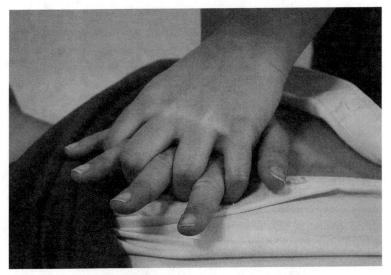

Figure 9.4 Interlock and extend the fingers

7. Compress the breastbone to a depth of 5–6cm (in adults) at a rate of 100-120 per minute. Following each compression, release the pressure, allowing the chest to completely recoil back to its pre-compression position (this will facilitate blood back to the heart). The compression and release phases should take equal amounts of time.

8. Perform chest compressions in a controlled manner; they should not be erratic or jerky.

9. Ensure chest compressions continued to be delivered at a rate of 100–120/min (this rate refers to the speed of compressions i.e. roughly 2 per second) rather than the actual number delivered per minute.

10. Ensure a ratio of 30 compressions: 2 ventilations (30:2) to allow more time for chest compressions.

11. To prevent fatigue, ideally rotate the rescuer performing chest compressions approximately every 2 minutes.

12. If not trained to, or unwilling to perform, mouth to mouth ventilation, perform chest compressions only at a rate of 100–120 per minute (see below).

Chest compressions-only CPR

If not trained to, or unwilling to, deliver rescue breaths, perform chest compressions only at a rate of 100–120 per minute (see compression-only CPR section below). This recommendation from the Resuscitation Council (UK) aims to increase the chances of a bystander performing CPR (if reluctant to perform mouth to mouth ventilation, bystanders may not perform CPR at all). Doing something is better than doing nothing.

Principles of mouth to mouth ventilation

Mouth to mouth ventilation is a quick, effective method to provide adequate oxygenation and ventilation in a casualty who is not breathing. However particular attention to the correct technique is essential. The most common cause of failure to ventilate is improper positioning of the head and chin.

Both healthcare workers and laypersons are often reluctant to perform mouth to mouth ventilation on a non-family member, usually because they fear contracting the HIV virus (there are no known cases of this happening). Consequently there are a variety of barrier devices available e.g. the simple face shield, which provide reassurance to the rescuer.

The procedure for mouth-mouth ventilation

1. Ensure the patient is flat on his back.
2. Kneel in a comfortable position with the knees a shoulder width apart, at the side of the patient at the level of his nose and mouth (a wider base will be required to undertake compressions if only one person performing CPR).
3. Rest back to sit on the heels in the low kneeling position (Resuscitation Council UK, 2001).
4. Apply a barrier device if one is available and if trained to use it.
5. Bend forwards from the hips leaning down towards the casualty's nose and mouth.
6. While maintaining head tilt and chin lift, use the index finger and thumb of the hand on the casualty's forehead to pinch the soft part his nose, open his mouth and take a normal breath in.
7. Place your lips around the casualty's mouth, ensure a good seal and blow into his mouth over 1 second, watching for chest rise.
8. While still maintaining head tilt and chin lift, remove your mouth and watch for chest fall. Repeat the procedure and then ensure another 30 chest compressions are performed. The delivery of two ventilations should take no longer than five seconds.

If rescue breaths do not achieve chest rise:

♦ Ensure adequate head tilt and chin lift

♦ Check the casualty's mouth and remove any obstruction

♦ Ensure a good seal between your mouth and the casualty's mouth

♦ Ensure the casualty's nose is pinched during ventilation

Automated external defibrillation

An automated external defibrillator (AED) (Fig. 9.5) can easily be used by a lay person, even without prior training.

AEDs are very simple and provide audio and/or visual instructions to the rescuer. They enable a casualty to be defibrillated by a bystander before the arrival of the ambulance service. To use an AED, switch it on and follow the instructions. Typically this will be:

1. Apply adhesive pad electrodes to the casualty's bare chest following the manufacturer's recommendations.

2. When the AED starts to analyse the ECG, stop CPR has instructed.

3. If shock is advised shout 'stand clear' and perform visual check to ensure no person is touching the patient before pressing the flashing shock button to shock the patient (Fig. 9.6) (if the AED is fully automated, it will deliver the shock automatically).

4. Continue CPR 30 compressions: 2 ventilations as guided by the voice/ visual prompts.

5. Following 2 minutes of CPR the AED will analyse the ECG again and a further shock will be advised if necessary.

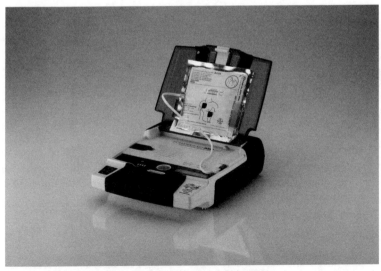

Figure 9.5 Example of automated external defibrillator (AED)

Reproduced with kind permission of Cardiac Science www.cardiacscience.com

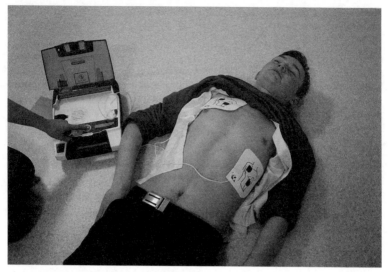

Figure 9.6 Automated external defibrillation

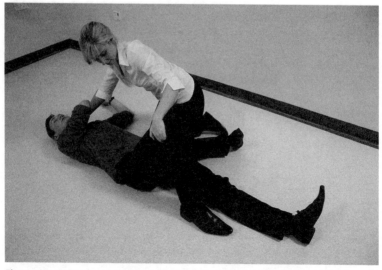

Figure 9.7 Grasp the casualty's far leg just above the knee and pull it up, taking care to keep the foot on the ground

The recovery position

If a person is unconscious (unresponsive) and lying on the back, the airway (the hollow passage that takes air to the lungs) can become blocked by the tongue falling backwards or by vomit if the casualty is sick.

Placing an unconscious casualty in the recovery position helps to keep the tongue forwards and reduces the risk of vomit entering the lungs if the casualty is sick. The recovery position is recommended if the casualty is unconscious, but breathing normally.

A suggested procedure for placing a casualty into the recovery position:

- ◆ Call out for help
- ◆ Ensure it is safe to approach
- ◆ Decide the best side to roll the casualty
- ◆ If necessary, remove spectacles and put them in a safe place

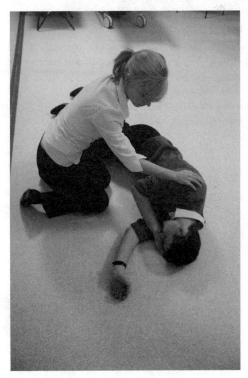

Figure 9.8 Recovery position

- Loosen any clothing around the neck

- Kneel beside the casualty, making sure the legs are straight

- Place the arm nearest to you at right angles to the casualty, with the elbow bent and palm of the hand upwards

- Grasp the far arm and bring it across his chest, holding the back of the hand against the casualty's cheek

- Using the free hand, grasp the casualty's far leg just above the knee and pull it up, taking care to keep the foot on the ground (Fig. 9.7)

- Whilst holding the casualty's hand against the cheek, pull on the far leg to roll the casualty towards you onto the side

- Adjust the upper leg, ensuring that both the hip and the knee are bent at right angles

- Tilt the head back to help ensure that the airway remains open. It may be necessary to adjust the hand under the casualty's cheek to help maintain this position (Fig. 9.8)

- If not already done, dial 999 (or 112) for an ambulance

- Regularly check that the casualty is still breathing normally

- If after 30 minutes the ambulance has not arrived, roll the casualty back onto the back and place in the recovery position on the other side.

Further reading and information

Current Resuscitation Council (UK) guidelines for resuscitation and defibrillation are available on www.resus.org.uk.

10

Further information on angina and heart attacks

Phil Jevon

A wealth of helpful information is available both locally and nationally. The British Heart Foundation remains one of the major sources of information relating to angina and heart attacks.

Local information

Heart related information is available from a number of local sources including:

♦ The patient's GP practice—e.g. GP, practice nurse, health visitor

♦ The local hospital's cardiac ward/coronary care unit e.g. cardiologist, ward sister, cardiac rehabilitation nurse and cardiac dietician

♦ The local cardiac rehabilitation centre

National information

There are many sources of information available nationally. The main source undoubtedly is the British Heart Foundation, but there are also other helpful sources.

British Heart Foundation

Head office: British heart Foundation

Greater London House

180 Hampstead Road

London NW1 7AW

Email: supporterservices@bhf.org.uk

Main telephone number: 020 7554 0000

Website: www.bhf.org.uk

Publications

A wide range of literature, DVDs, podcasts, etc are available on all topics related to angina and heart attacks. Many are available in ethnic languages as well.

British Heart Foundation's Heart Telephone HelpLine

The British Heart Foundation's Heart Telephone Helpline is designed to help both patients and carers by providing information, support and guidance on heart related matters. The helpline is staffed by cardiac nurses and heart health advisors.

The telephone number is 0300 330 3311. Lines are open 9am–5pm Monday–Friday.

Email queires are also possible via an on-line contact us form.

British Heart Foundation's audio podcasts

A number of cardiac themed podcasts are available to download from http://www.bhf.org.uk/community/our-podcasts.aspx

◆ Alcohol and your heart

◆ Chest pain and heart attacks

◆ Risk factors and heart disease

◆ Heart drugs and you

◆ Managing weight

◆ Understanding heart conditions

◆ Blood pressure and your heart

◆ Cholesterol and how to control it

◆ Holidays, travel insurance and your heart

◆ Recovery with a heart condition

◆ Smoking and how to give up

British Heart Foundation's video podcast

A video podcast on cardiac rehabilitation is available on http://www.bhf.org.uk/community/our-podcasts.aspx

Watch Your Own heart attack video

The British Heart Foundation has produced a two-minute video called Watch Your Own Heart Attack starring the actor Steven Berkoff. It is available to watch on www.youtube.com - type in *watch your own heart attack*.

British Heart Foundations' Heart Information Series

The British Heart Foundation has published 25 booklets in its Heart Information Series on a variety of cardiac related topics including angina, heart attack and coronary angioplasty. These are available to download from www.bhf.org.uk or they can be ordered from the BHF orderline: 0870 600 6566.

Stopping Smoking – Further Information

NHS stop smoking services

The NHS stop smoking service provides a wealth of information relating to stopping smoking. Its website provides helpful information including how to quit and local NHS stop smoking services.

It is produced a Quit Kit which has been compiled based on advice from experts, smokers and ex-smokers. It is packed with practical tools and advice to help you quit smoking for good. It also includes a voucher for a week's free trial of Nicotine Replacement Therapy (NRT) patches, which can double the chances of quitting successfully compared to willpower alone.

Contact details:

NHS Free Smoking Helpline: 0800 022 4 332 Mon to Fri 9am to 8pm, Sat and Sun 11am to 5pm

www.smokefree.nhs.uk

QUIT

The aim of QUIT is to:

◆ Significantly reduce unnecessary suffering and death from smoking related diseases

◆ Aim towards a smoke free UK future

◆ Provide practical help, advice and support by trained counsellors to all smokers who want to stop.

Contact details:

QUIT

63 St. Marys Axe

London EC3A 8AA

T: 0207 469 0400

F: 0207 469 0401

info@quit.org.uk

Resuscitation

Resuscitation Council UK

The objective of the Council is to facilitate education of both lay and healthcare professional members of the population in the most effective methods of resuscitation appropriate to their needs.

Resuscitation guidelines are available, including helpful flow charts and background information.

Resuscitation Council (UK)

5th Floor

Tavistock House North

Tavistock Square

London WC1H 9HR

Telephone: 020 7388 4678

Fax: 020 7383 0773

Website: www.resus.org.uk

Index